The Four Dragons

The Four Dragons

Clearing the Meridians and Awakening the Spine in Nei Gong

DAMO MITCHELL

FOREWORD BY DR OLE SAETHER

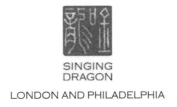

SINGING
DRAGON

LONDON AND PHILADELPHIA

First published in 2014
by Singing Dragon
an imprint of Jesscia Kingsley Publishers
73 Collier Street
London N1 9BE, UK
and
400 Market Street, Suite 400
Philadelphia, PA 19106, USA

www.singingdragon.com

Library of Congress Cataloging in Publication Data
Mitchell, Damo.
The four dragons : clearing the meridians and awakening
the spine in nei gong / Damo Mitchell ;
foreword by Dr. Ole Saether.
pages cm
Includes index.
ISBN 978-1-84819-226-3 (alk. paper)
1. Dao yin. 2. Qi gong. 3. Back exercises. I. Title.
RA781.85.M58 2014
613.7'1489--dc23
2014004432

British Library Cataloguing in Publication Data
A CIP catalogue record for this book is available from the British Library

ISBN 978 1 84819 226 3
eISBN 978 0 85701 173 2

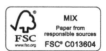

MIX
Paper from
responsible sources
FSC
www.fsc.org   FSC® C013604

To my parents and friends,
Paul and Chris

Contents

FOREWORD

I first met Damo in Stockholm in March 2012, during one of his workshops on Daoist Nei Gong. What really struck me about Damo was his incredible flexibility and his speed of movement, as well as the ease with which he taught. Daoist theory just seemed to come to him very naturally – and so did his explanations, his practical demonstrations and his Qi transmission. During the course, he went through different practices, including stretching, Zhan Zhuang (standing stake) and Qi Gong. He also helped us awaken our energy system.

I had decided to attend this workshop mainly for health reasons. Prior to training with Damo, I had trained in Yi Quan/Taikkiken and this had proven to be great for my health. My teacher had helped me out with the Zhan Zhuang posture, which I found rather tricky at first. This standing practice actually cured the chronic muscular pain from which I had been suffering for the previous twenty years. But then, all of a sudden, the training gave me pain in my lower back. The more I trained the more pain I experienced, especially at night when I wasn't moving.

I made all sorts of adjustments to my Yi Quan training but nothing helped, so I had to stop training. I went to see four different acupuncturists, to no avail unfortunately; the fourth one actually made it worse as he caused some psychological disturbances! The fifth acupuncturist I met was my TCM (Traditional Chinese Medicine) teacher. He was also a very good chiropractor and he found out that there was something wrong with my right sacro-iliac joint. Things improved after this adjustment. However, the tension in my lower back wouldn't go away, even after a few more acupuncture treatments.

Before receiving the treatment from my acupuncture teacher, I had been searching for workshops that could potentially help me. I had just finished reading *Daoist Nei Gong* – Damo's first book – and, to my surprise, it turned out that Damo was about to visit Stockholm in March 2012. I didn't know what to expect when I went to that workshop; but I have been following Damo's teachings since then and I feel very lucky that our paths crossed. I have learned various practices with Damo, including Ji Ben Qi Gong, Wu Xing Qi Gong and the Dragon Dao Yin exercises, as well as meditation. Although I have only studied the Dragon Dao Yin sequences for a year now, they have made my body much softer and more flexible.

Who may benefit from this book then? I would say that if you are following Damo's teachings, the book is essential because it will speed up the understanding of the system and make the Dragon Dao Yin exercises come to life much faster. For those training in other systems like Qi Gong or yoga, it is also a very valuable book because it explains the difference between Qi Gong and Dao Yin exercises. The book goes through the Dao Yin sequences in detail. As an added benefit, the Dragon Dao Yin might be helpful to yoga practitioners, as they open the joints. Just as important, the book provides a comprehensive theoretical overview of Dao Yin and Qi Gong.

When it comes to this type of training, people often worry about a number of things. How much time should I spend on this training? Is there really something called Qi in the body? Is this good for my health? What is the purpose of this Daoist training? If we wish to understand what Damo teaches, it is required that we put some time into it.

Unlike Western medicine, Chinese medicine rests on the idea that everything is Qi. Damo teaches through the ancient Chinese way of looking at the world and understanding the energies that surround us. It isn't easy to find teachers who have such in-depth knowledge. It is also very hard to find someone who speaks English and is actually willing to teach Western people. For these reasons, Damo's books are, in my opinion, as rare as they are unique.

While Nei Gong training is really good for your health, this is ultimately a by-product of the training. The meaning of the training is to try and understand Dao. But what Dao exactly is, no one knows. It is just a big question mark.

Welcome to a journey on the road into the unknown…

Dr Ole Saether
Doctor of Western medicine, Chinese medicine
practitioner and Nei Gong practitioner
Gothenburg, Sweden

ACKNOWLEDGEMENTS

First and foremost, thank you to my good friend Spencer Hill for working so hard to create the amazing drawings used to demonstrate the movements of the Dragon Dao Yin exercises. Thanks also to Joe Andrews for the line drawings used elsewhere in the book. Much gratitude to the students featured in photographs in this book: Jason Smith and Tom Burrows. Thank you to Dr Ole Saether for kindly writing the foreword to this book. Thank you so much to Linda Griffiths who provided the photo of the dragon chasing the pearl for me. Last but not least, thanks once again to Jessica Kingsley and the staff at Singing Dragon for allowing my ramblings to make it into print once more.

Disclaimer

The author and publisher of this material are not responsible in any way whatsoever for any injury that may occur through reading or practising the exercises outlined in this book.

The exercises and practices may be too strenuous or risky for some people and so you should consult a qualified doctor before attempting anything from this book. It is also advised that you proceed under the guidance of an experienced teacher of the internal arts to avoid injury and confusion.

Note that no form of internal exercise is a substitute for conventional health practices, medicines or any form of psychotherapy.

NOTES ON THE TEXT

Throughout this book I have used the Pinyin system of Romanisation for the majority of Chinese words. Please note that much of the theory in this book differs greatly from Western science. The classical Chinese approach to understanding the organs of the body, for example, is based around the function of their energetic system rather than their physical anatomy. To distinguish the two understandings from each other I used capitalisation to indicate the Chinese understanding of the term. 'Heart' refers to the classical Chinese understanding of the organ, whilst 'heart' refers to the physical organ as understood in contemporary Western biological sciences.

PREFACE

The first time I encountered the Dragon Dao Yin exercises was a number of years ago in Shandong, north-east China. There are a lot of martial arts practitioners in Shandong and I would say that there are more people practising the internal arts in the parks early in the morning there than in many of the other provinces that I have visited.

I had originally come to Shandong to study an interesting variant of the Chen style of Taijiquan but alongside this I ended up learning from other teachers there as well. The Dragon Dao Yin exercises were a part of this extra study. They were originally taken from the Baguazhang martial arts style, as students there worked through the movements (mainly the walks) in order to soften the various muscles required for their forms training and get the spine ready for the demanding workout it has to go through during the early days of Bagua training. From this training it was seen just how effective the exercises were at conditioning the spine and so they gradually became adapted into a health exercise as well; though divorced from the martial principles and slightly adapted, it is still clear to see some of the movements of Baguazhang in the Dragon Dao Yin postures.

Training the walking exercises was a lot of fun as I joined not only the morning Bagua training but also the medical Dragon Dao Yin group to work on strengthening my spine. Most of those going through the exercises in the morning were much older than me and mostly Chinese women, so I stood out like a sore thumb, walking up and down twisting my body each day. I was especially put to shame by some of the more elderly members of the group who regularly liked to show me up by dropping into low splits and the most demanding Dao Yin postures with ease. To be honest, I think I was something of a novelty to the group, something of a mascot to show off to passers-by, but I did not mind; I liked my 'grandmotherly' classmates and enjoyed the morning training.

When I first started teaching the Dragon Dao Yin exercises I was surprised by just how effective they were. Many of my students had been working on standing postures, moving Qi Gong exercises and countless stretches in order to improve their posture, but just one day of the first two Dragon Dao Yin exercises was enough to do the job. There were lots of clicks and cracks that day as bones moved and bodies opened up. Since this time I have taught the Dragon Dao Yin exercises in the UK, Sweden and the US, and each time students have enjoyed the dynamic nature of the exercises and reported a great many health benefits. Though I still use these exercises as body conditioning for Baguazhang, they primarily form part of my medical exercise repertoire and the majority of students in my school know the movements and practise them as part of their regular routine.

In 2011 I released a small self-published book that mainly included photographs showing the various movements. It was originally intended as a visual aid for those learning the exercises from me, but despite this I received messages from around the world saying how much people were enjoying 'distance learning' the sequences from me and how much their health had benefited from the practice. The book was adequate for learning the movements but lacking in any depth, with no theoretical basis for what people were doing. For this reason I decided to rewrite the entire book from scratch with a great deal of the information students would need in order to understand exactly how the exercises worked. This book is the finished product, with the photographs replaced with excellent hand-drawn images that are much easier to follow.

I have introduced the basic theory which underlines the practice of Dao Yin training in general, before moving on to the exercises themselves which enable students to begin to put these principles into practice. From here I have moved on to some of the more complex aspects of working with these exercises and the energies of the spine. Namely this includes the generally misunderstood process of 'Waking up the Dragon' and the progression to more advanced Nei Dan training. These are difficult areas to discuss as when these stages are reached we are essentially working with something so ethereal it is difficult to tie down to an actual location in either the physical or the energy body. I have done my best though, and combined theory with my own rather limited experiences of working at these stages, so please show some understanding as I clumsily stumble my way through explaining the more esoteric aspects of the practice!

Though a book or video is never a substitute for hands-on teaching, I am confident that those who persevere will be able to work their way carefully through the instructions in the book and learn the Dragon Dao Yin sequences. I am happy to have had the opportunity to teach so many people the exercises contained in this book and I hope you enjoy learning the Dragon Dao Yin...

Damo Mitchell
Hong Kong
December 2013

CHAPTER 1

AN INTRODUCTION TO DAO YIN AND HEALTH

Prior to the formation of Daoism as a systemised tradition there lived the shamanic Wu people. With a history stretching back into antiquity, exact details about their practices are few and far between. Mythological stories and ancient writings tell tales of a group who served as healers, mystics and spiritual guides to the small nomadic communities that made up Chinese society at this time. These early practitioners of the energetic arts are recognised as the forefathers of practices such as Chinese medicine, astrology and even callisthenic exercises that would later go on to form Qi Gong and the internal martial arts.

The development of Qi Gong thus went through various periods of change and adjustment as the beliefs and understandings of the people practising them changed. Excavated tombs such as the recent treasure trove of archaeological findings uncovered at the Mawangdui dig[1] have enabled us to glimpse more clearly how these changes took place. One such development was the change of emphasis that took place from Dao Yin to Qi Gong exercises. The term Dao Yin is generally understood to be much older than the term Qi Gong and many theorists believe that these two terms are interchangeable; this is not my belief and in this book I aim to outline the qualitative differences between Qi Gong and Dao Yin so that those practising the internal arts may better utilise the two different practice modalities in order to assist in their internal development.

In order to understand the difference between Dao Yin and Qi Gong it is wise to look at the nature of the difference between the shamanic Wu people and the alchemical Daoists who appeared much later.

---

1   Mawangdui is an archaeological site located in Changsha, China. The site contained the tombs of three people from the western Han Dynasty. Many classical texts were found in one of the tombs, including depictions of Dao Yin exercises.

The Wu people were worshippers of the land. Historical evidence shows that, like most ancient cultures on earth, the Wu venerated the spirit of the planet, the elements, the weather, the animals and the energy of life that permeates all living things. Their study was an attempt at understanding the position which mankind took in the great cycle of life. Ancient practices such as circle-walking, star stepping and other ritualistic dances seem to have their roots in the practices of these ancient people. In short, though they may well have had a deep understanding of the inner workings of the human consciousness, the majority of their practices were 'outwards' in nature. Sickness was seen as the result of unwanted entities entering the body; misfortune was due to unhappiness amongst the spirits that governed the earth, and cures for these ills involved appeasement of the spirits.

Whilst it is true that many of these beliefs are still strong in Daoism and the arts that are heavily influenced by the philosophy of the Dao, such as Chinese medicine, there was a major shift at some point towards 'inward' focused practices. The major change came with the development of alchemical theory which, once again, started externally with the ingestion of various substances but then gradually shifted towards a search for the immortal elixir based around internal, energetic substances. Whilst the basic understanding of humankind being an integral part of the wider environment was still present, there was now more study taking place of the nature of the human microcosm.

In ancient writings we see the term Dao Yin appearing as early as Chinese written records. Ancient scrolls such as the Dao Yin Tu show that these were being practised in at least 2000 BC and almost certainly much earlier. References to Dao Yin training appear in many classical texts including such influential pieces such as the *Huang Di Nei Jing* and the *Chuang Tzu*; these references appeared much earlier than the term Qi Gong, which most people in the internal arts community are familiar with today.

Dao Yin exercises are discussed in terms of the key words: stretching, expelling, leading and guiding. The last two terms, 'leading' and 'guiding', are a direct translation of the Chinese term Dao Yin. The Chinese characters Dao Yin are shown in Figure 1.1.

The aim of these stretching exercises was to purge stagnant energy from the body, which, classically, was seen as the result of evil spirits, or negative environmental energies invading us from the outside. The emphasis of Dao Yin exercises was therefore on the outer world. Sickness developed primarily from an external source and now, through opening the body and guiding the negative Qi out, this sickness was pushed back into the outside world.

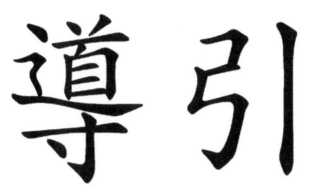

FIGURE 1.1: DAO YIN CHARACTERS

In contrast to this, Qi Gong exercises were formed later when understandings had changed. Although it was still believed that negative influences could come from our environment there was more of a study of our own inner nature and how it affected us. Alchemical teachings, along with the philosophy of realised human beings such as Lao Tzu, showed that sickness could come from inside as well through the effects of our own mind. Stagnation was seen as the key enemy, along with the concept of deficient or excessive energetic qualities, and the emphasis was more on internal practices. Although Qi Gong still purges toxins from the energy system, it primarily works to nourish and regulate our already existing energy. The movements tend to be gentler, the mind is kept inside (most of the time) and the aim is rarely to push out into the environment.

These qualitative differences really distinguish Dao Yin and Qi Gong from each other, although they share common elements due to Qi Gong being developed from Dao Yin training. Confusion comes in modern times when different teachers use different terminology. One of the first challenges when studying under a new teacher is learning exactly how they use the terminology to describe what they are doing. Essentially it does not really matter. Terminology is just that, a way of labelling something; it is the practice itself that matters, but at the same time it can be useful to understand what quality an individual style of exercise is supposed to have. According to my own definitions there are actually many groups practising Dao Yin, which they call Qi Gong, and vice versa.

I believe that it is useful to be able to understand and practise both forms of exercise as distinct entities in their own right. The exercises that we use are only tools in order to move through a process, a process of internal growth, development and understanding. This process of change is classically known as Nei Gong and moving through it requires that we do not see the exercises themselves as the end goal. Once we become fixated on simply repeating the various movements we have learnt without any larger direction, then we cease to develop. Our practice has resulted in stagnation, which will not lead us towards any state of realisation. As we move along the path to Dao, the path of Nei Gong, we must understand how to use our different tools at the correct times and in the correct manner in order to keep progressing. Sometimes I believe the more Yang Dao Yin exercises are more suitable, whilst at other times it is wisest to focus upon the more Yin Qi Gong exercises we have learnt.

One teacher explained stagnation in the body to me as being like rust blocking up the pipes in a radiator system. The rust which has built up will prevent water from flowing effectively, which will then lead to problems; this is like stuck Qi in our meridian system. If we use Qi Gong to dissolve this rust then water will be able to flow once more, restoring health to some degree, but essentially the rust is still in the system. If, however, we are able to actually purge the rust from the radiator pipes then water will flow once more and there is little chance of that rust building up again. Dao Yin is a method that aims to clear rust from the system through its emphasis on purging into the external environment. Does that make Dao Yin superior? Not at all, it just means it is more suitable for that particular purpose. Qi Gong is far more efficient for making sure things run smoothly after this purging has taken place.

Table 1.1 summarises the key qualitative differences between Dao Yin and Qi Gong training.

TABLE 1.1: KEY DIFFERENCES BETWEEN QI GONG AND DAO YIN

	Qi Gong Exercises	Dao Yin Exercises
Polarity	Yin	Yang
Key aims	Nourishing and regulating	Purging
Bodywork	Soft and gentle	Soft and stretched
Pathway utilised	Meridians	Jing Jin pathways
Co-ordination	Simple	More complex
Breathing	Yin abdominal	Yang abdominal
Intention	In (generally)	Outside
General function	To build up	To cleanse

POLARITY

Generally Qi Gong exercises tend to be far more Yin in quality than Dao Yin exercises, which are generally far more Yang. The overall feel from Qi Gong exercises is far more calming and brings a practitioner closer to a point of inner stillness than Dao Yin training, which can stir up a great deal of internal movement. Qi Gong would approach the subject of inner cultivation from the more subtle direction of mental stillness, whilst Dao Yin exercises seek to cultivate through activity and excitement.

KEY PRINCIPLES

Qi Gong exercises generally work to nourish a practitioner's energy body with fresh Qi, which is drawn from the air and from the Earth's Qi which moves up through the legs. This Qi is then circulated through the various elements of the energy body, ensuring that any imbalances are regulated. Dao Yin exercises still accomplish this to a lesser extent but they primarily serve to expel pathogenic Qi from the body via one or more key exit points, which are discussed later in this book; this is the process of purging which is the key aim of Dao Yin. Earth Qi entering the body in Qi Gong tends to be directed towards circulation, whilst the planets' Qi drawn up through Dao Yin exercises is directed straight through the body and out into the distance, turning the body into an energetic conduit. It is this 'flowing through' which serves to clear pathogenic Qi from the body.

BODYWORK

Qi Gong exercises generally (but not always) use very soft, gentle movements which are rhythmic, relaxed and led by soft breathing. Very little force is used so that the Qi may flow smoothly through the meridians, which run primarily through the layers of fascia in the body. Dao Yin exercises are still relaxed but they are generally more 'stretched out' in nature. The joints are opened and the various layers of the physical body are lengthened so that Qi may be moved through the body much like toothpaste being gently squeezed through a tube. In this way Dao Yin exercises have a lot in common with the yogic exercises of India; it is for this reason that you will often find them referred to as Daoist yoga, which is a modern term rather than a classical one.

PATHWAY UTILISED

Qi Gong exercises generally aim to move Qi information along the line of the meridians; at first this will be the acquired meridians which are closely linked to the organs of the body, but at higher stages this Qi flow will move in the congenital meridian pathways. Dao Yin exercises also move Qi in the meridians but this takes place as a by-product of working with the Jing Jin pathways of connective tissue. By stretching and lengthening the Jing Jin pathways they have a directional effect upon the meridians, which then pass Qi out from the body. The Jing Jin pathways are discussed in detail in Chapter 2. The only exception to this is at an advanced level where the congenital meridians may be engaged. An example of this would be an advanced process like 'Waking up the Dragon', which is discussed in Chapter 7 of this book.

CO-ORDINATION

Qi Gong exercises are generally fairly simple to learn. Dao Yin exercises can be a little more complex, with more exact body movement principles to ensure that the various joints of the body are effectively opened and the pathways for the Qi are positioned so that Qi may efficiently be expelled. It is also more common to twist and stretch the body in Dao Yin. The spine is often pumped and opened out, which can be more demanding than the bodywork found in the majority of Qi Gong systems.

BREATHING

There are many different breathing techniques in the Daoist internal tradition. For most of the time when people are practising Qi Gong exercises they are using deep abdominal breathing patterns. There may be variations upon this technique but in the majority of cases these techniques fall in the abdominal breathing category. Experience has shown that this is the most effective and safest way to circulate Qi through the body. Yin abdominal breathing methods use a gentle expansion and then passive contraction of the abdominal muscles and intercostal muscles in order to allow Qi to circulate smoothly and naturally through the body. Dao Yin exercises tend to use more Yang abdominal breathing patterns. These differ from the Yin methods in placing more emphasis on the process of exhaling to lead Qi to a desired location (usually out of the body). Yang abdominal breathing is discussed in Chapter 4 of this book.

INTENTION

Most Qi Gong practices require that the practitioner places their awareness either in the body or close to the body, often near to their palms. This is conducive to leading the Qi to the ideal location for reinforcing the nourishing and regulating function of that particular exercise. Dao Yin exercises usually require the intention to be far from the body and out into the distance. This makes it much easier for stagnant Qi to begin being purged. As a general rule, if we want our Qi to move an inch we need about a metre of extension of our intention. For this reason it is generally advisable to have as much distance in front of you as possible when you practise, in order to fully extend the intention.

GENERAL FUNCTION

Most Qi Gong exercises, from the medical tradition, aim to 'build up' a person. Fresh Qi is brought into the body so that any deficiencies are taken care of and energy levels are improved along with whatever regulating functions that particular exercise is designed to perform. Dao Yin exercises may still do this to some degree but they are primarily designed to 'cleanse' the meridian system of stagnant energies. They also help to open the joints to a higher degree, helping the body to loosen up.

ENERGY GATES

In order to understand how Dao Yin exercises work we must first have an understanding of the various aspects of both the physical and the energetic body that are involved in Dao Yin training. Key areas of the energy body known as Qi Men are heavily involved in Dao Yin practice, and it is with these that we are aiming to work.

Stagnant Qi sits largely in the body's joints. In each of our joints there are numerous energetic pathways which the Daoists call Qi Men or 'energy gates'. The meridian system runs throughout our entire body ensuring a healthy flow of Qi to all of our organs and tissues. The flow of Qi in the meridian system is dependent on several factors, including a healthy lower Dan Tien, a good posture and a high level of 'potential difference', which will assist Qi with flowing from an area of high resistance to an area of low resistance. As our bodies move and we naturally stretch and compress the pathways of the meridian system, as well as the more physical pathways of the Jing Jin (lines of connective tissue), potential difference alternates and so Qi flows steadily around our body. The 'energy gates' are the points that divide the body into areas of high and low resistance.

If a person maintains a healthy degree of movement and good posture throughout their life, then the chances are that their 'energy gates' will remain open and Qi will flow freely. Sadly, the majority of people in modern times do not maintain a healthy level of exercise and good posture. This means that the degree of 'potential difference' is low and the energy gates become compressed by misalignment of the bones. Qi will now collect in the joints and stagnation occurs. Over time, stagnation leads to major blockages, tightness and finally sickness.

Dao Yin exercises are designed to gently pull open the joints and realign the bones so as to prevent illness from taking hold. This is the meaning of the character Yin 引 ('to lead'). The focused use of mental intention then directs pathogens out through the pathway which has been opened; this is the meaning of the character Dao 導 ('to guide').

It is important in our training that we keep in mind the location of the key energy gates in our body and maintain a gentle pull on them when we practise. This pull should be just enough for it to feel as though our body is being gently 'teased' open in this area. Note that forceful stretching is actually counterproductive as it will lead to tension and thus further stagnation. Figure 1.2 shows the location of the key energy gates that are utilised in the majority of Dao Yin exercises.

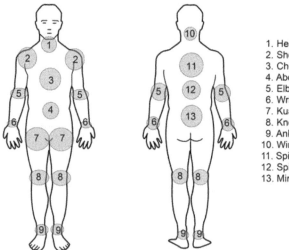

1. Heavenly Prominence Gate
2. Shoulder Nest Gates
3. Chest Centre Gate
4. Abdominal Gate
5. Elbow Gates
6. Wrist Gates
7. Kua Gates
8. Knee Gates
9. Ankle Gates
10. Wind Palace Gate
11. Spirit Path Gate
12. Spine Centre Gate
13. Ming Men Gate

FIGURE 1.2: MAJOR QI MEN (ENERGY GATES)

Minor energy gates also exist in the body and sit in every space between our bones, from the joints of our fingers and toes to the plates which make up our skull. The first stage in Dao Yin training with regard to the energy gates is the opening of the major gates. The next stage is systematically working through all of the minor gates. If we can achieve this then we are bringing a healthy flow of Qi into and out of the body as we breathe; our body will become an energetic conduit for the Qi of the environment, and so we can be said to have achieved 'energetic emptiness' according to the ancient Daoists.

Throughout the body we have numerous energetic pathways through which our body's Qi flows; collectively these are known as the Jing Luo, the meridian system. Running like a superhighway of information throughout the body, the meridian system governs the vital functions of the organs and systems of the body, at the same time as enabling living creatures to communicate energetically with the powers of Heaven and Earth. It is through the meridian system that our inner consciousness communicates with the physical world, forming the mind–body link that is all-important in Daoism. These are the same energetic pathways as those utilised in therapeutic practices such as shiatsu and acupuncture or internal practices such as Heavenly Streams practice. Traditionally, students of Daoism would learn to connect with and feel their meridian system before practising any Chinese medicine (see my previous book, *Heavenly Streams*,[2] which describes how this type of skill can be developed). Figure 1.3 shows the layout of the meridian system.

As shown in Figure 1.3, the meridians flow through the entire body, including the joints where the energy gates sit. Many of the most powerful meridian points utilised in Chinese medicine sit in these joints and their function relies upon their connection to the energy gates located in this area of the body. Qi is a form of vibratory information which carries conscious information throughout the body (for a further discussion of this concept please refer to my previous book *Daoist Nei Gong: The Philosophical Art of Change*[3]), but for the purposes of understanding its ebbs and flows we can return to the metaphor of water. If Qi flows like water through the body, then when it reaches the joints it pools, and indeed many meridian points located in the body's joints are named after pools, ponds and even oceans. A combination of our breath, the force of the Dan Tien rotating (which

2   Mitchell, D. (2013) *Heavenly Streams: Meridian Theory in Nei Gong*. London: Singing Dragon.

3   Mitchell, D. (2011) *Daoist Nei Gong: The Philosophical Art of Change*. London: Singing Dragon.

is discussed in Chapter 7) and bodily movement ensures that the water continues to flow and so harmony is maintained. Problems arise if one of two things happens:

1. The joints are not moved regularly. Inactivity means that the Qi is not shifted by the potential difference created through movement of the body's joints. The 'pumping' function of the joint is not taking place and so stagnation begins to set in.

2. Injury, sickness or tension tightens the body. If the body tightens then the muscles and tissues around the joints contract, resulting in a 'closed' joint. This restricts the Qi in the energy gates, meaning that stagnation occurs.

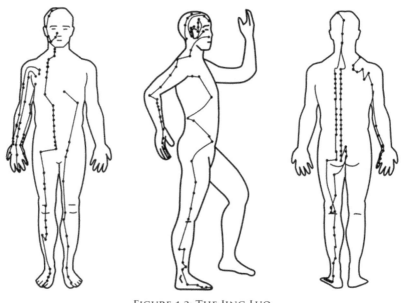

FIGURE 1.3: THE JING LUO

Within the Daoist tradition stagnation is always a negative thing, as stagnant energy begins to fester. Like a festering pool, the quality of the Qi is greatly lessened and this will gradually lead to the development of sickness. From this we can see that Dao Yin exercises aim to open the joints and keep them moving healthily in order to prevent this from happening.

An important factor often missed when studying the nature of the energy gates is their connection to the movement of Qi through different layers of depth in the energy body. The meridian system works to connect our inner universe to the outer universe in which we live. Qi from the outside moves in towards our core and at the same time our energy body shifts energy from inside to outside of our body. In this way our energetic system 'breathes' Qi in the same way as our lungs breathe air. Through the pores of the skin external Qi enters the body where it moves through the Jing Jin and surface meridians until it reaches the joints of the body; from here some of this energy moves deeper into the body. Figure 1.4 shows the movement of Qi as we breathe.

This energetic form of 'respiration' which takes place during our practice assists in moving pathogenic factors from deep inside the body out towards the surface of the body, where they can be cleared. There are also strong exit points on the body which we can utilise to increase the efficiency of the purging process, and the Dragon Dao Yin exercises make good use of these points.

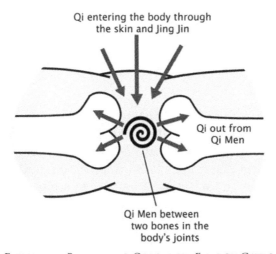

FIGURE 1.4: BREATHING QI VIA THE ENERGY GATES

There are many points upon the energy body which can be used to expel pathogens from the body but in general we use the following points in Dao Yin training: Laogong (PC 8) and the Shixuan points (Extra points), one of which is Zhongchong (PC 9), actually the strongest of the Shixuan points, situated in the tip of the middle finger. Figure 1.5 shows the location of these points.

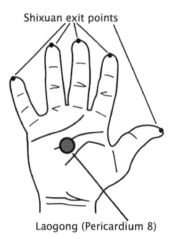

Shixuan exit points

Laogong (Pericardium 8)

FIGURE 1.5: KEY EXIT POINTS

In Dao Yin training we generally aim to lead pathogens out towards these points. Numerous other points on the energy body are utilised in Dao Yin training, and these are discussed at relevant stages in this book.

THE DAO OF HEALTH

The Daoist view of health is threefold. According to this ancient school of thought we must maintain the health of our physical body, energy body and consciousness in order to prevent the development of disease. To achieve this we must learn to live with and harness the energy of our environment. This is the traditional way to achieve union with the great creative force of Dao, which will in turn lead to the elevation of consciousness.

Our physical body must be kept healthy, as this is the vehicle through which we experience existence. Yang Sheng Fa (life-nourishing techniques) was the study of the health of the physical body. Traditionally Yang Sheng Fa included teachings on maintaining a correct and healthy diet, breathing exercises, physical exercises such as Dao Yin, and Chinese medicine such as the study of herbs and self-massage.

The physical body's health provides the foundation for well-being on an energetic level, which in turn helps to build the health of your consciousness. Quite simply it is our physical health that must be worked on first. We cannot fall into the trap of working solely on the energy body whilst ignoring the physical body, a trap which many energy workers unfortunately fall into.

The Daoist view of physical health is quite different from the traditional view of physical health according to Western thought. In the West we often view the healthy male body as being immensely strong with a broad muscular chest and large biceps. The Daoist view is that this sort of figure is damaging to your health, as all of your muscles and tendons have been shortened and tightened. This tightness leads to stagnation which manifests within the physical, energetic and consciousness body. The 'healthy' female body in the West is equally incorrect according to the Daoist tradition, which would view the stick-like figure of a supermodel as a sign of severe deficiency. Internal artists should aim to keep their bodies slim (but not thin), with a good level of flexibility, mobile joints, good posture and good core strength. People should not worry about gaining a little extra weight around the area of the kidneys and midriff as they get older, as this helps to preserve the kidneys' health, but excessive weight is definitely seen as negative. An excess of body weight is not healthy according to Daoist thought. There is an idea within many contemporary Daoist schools that being overweight and having a large belly is a sign of internal development. This is quite simply not true; the concept of the 'Qi belly' is a myth. It is true that prolonged abdominal breathing will cause your abdominal muscles to relax and leave you with a slight 'pot belly' after many years, but this is definitely different from the belly that develops through inactivity, excessive food and too much alcohol.

NEGATIVE OR PATHOGENIC QI

The Qi that flows within your meridian system can have either a good or bad influence on your health depending on whether it is positive or negative. Quite simply, we want to increase the amount of positive Qi that flows through us and expel any negative Qi that leads to stagnation.

Qi takes the form of a vibrational wave which you can feel moving in the body once you have trained for a sufficient time. The Qi vibration carries information through your body in a similar way to binary code providing the information for computer systems. It comprises peaks and troughs, or Yin and Yang as the ancient Daoists called it. The various combinations of Yin and Yang waves create different bundles of information, which in turn lead to various energetic movements. The Daoists mapped out these energetic movements in a text known as the *Yi Jing* (Classic of Changes); they represented them diagrammatically, as shown in Figure 1.6.

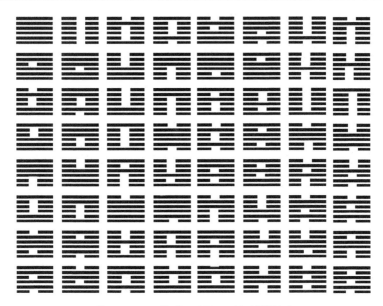

FIGURE 1.6: QI INFORMATION WAVES

These groups of information are known as 'hexagrams'. A person trained in the use of the *Yi Jing* can use it to determine the likelihood and nature of change in the environment, or as a diagnostic tool that can help to understand illness in the complex network of the human energy body.

Our Qi reacts with the energy of the environment, other people and our own consciousness which is constantly sending information from our mind into our energy system. If any of this information is negative in content, then it can adversely affect the quality of the Qi flowing within us. The nature of this negative or pathogenic Qi is divided into two main categories: internal and external. Internal pathogens are negative forms of Qi generated by emotions, past psychological trauma, a poor diet or a poor-quality lifestyle. External pathogens are considered to be due to environmental pathogens or physical trauma. For a further discussion of these please refer to my previous book, *Heavenly Streams: Meridian Theory in Nei Gong*.

External pathogenic Qi moves from outside our body, through the superficial layers of the energy system and then progressively deeper into the body. Internal pathogenic Qi is already in our core and gradually begins to manifest in the comparatively exterior layers of our energetic and physical body. In practice, the actual nature of the pathogenic Qi is not that important as it all needs expelling from the body, and so it must all move from our centre out towards the surface where we can conduct it towards one of our main exit points.

In the case of internal pathogenic Qi developed from an emotional source, the ancient Daoists were able to map out correlations between physical locations in the body and psychological states. Through centuries of experiential learning they began to find patterns between where the Qi would settle and stagnate and what was going on for a person emotionally. For example, people who are unable to let go of some past sadness will often find that the resultant internal pathogenic Qi sits in the area of the meridian system that governs the functioning of the lungs. For this reason, sadness and grief are linked with the lungs in Chinese medicine. Particular meridian points could then be identified in therapies such as acupuncture as being useful in the treatment of lung weakness, as they affect any pathogenic Qi stagnating in this part of the energy body. (Please note that these correlations do not directly apply to pathogenic factors originating outside the body, as here the process of stagnation is different.) It is worth looking at the link between bodily locations of stagnant pathogenic Qi and psychological states, as the vast majority of people's poor energetic and physical health is a direct result of their emotional state. Where there is stagnant pathogenic Qi there will be physical discomfort, tightness, pain or even organ weakness. Figure 1.7 shows the different areas of the body which become painful due to pathogenic Qi.

Although this theory is a very general way of understanding the negative mind–body link it is good enough to give you an understanding of why you may have tightness, pain or discomfort in various regions of your body.

Since, in the author's experience, the vast majority of energetic stagnations are due to emotional disturbances, a large section of this book has been dedicated to the study of internally based pathogens. Although it is likely that the original shamanic nature of Dao Yin exercises focused largely upon externally based pathogens, experience has shown that they are very powerful tools for clearing stagnant energy left from past psychological trauma and habitual emotional patterns.

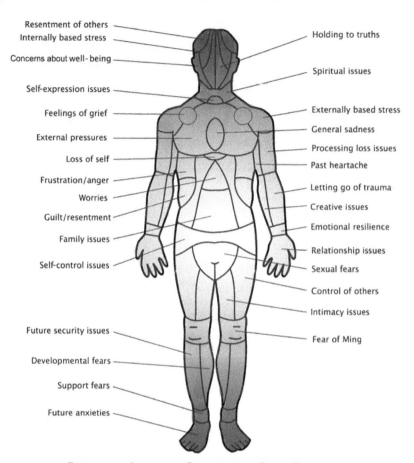

Resentment of others
Internally based stress
Concerns about well- being
Self-expression issues
Feelings of grief
External pressures
Loss of self
Frustration/anger
Worries
Guilt/resentment
Family issues
Self-control issues
Future security issues
Developmental fears
Support fears
Future anxieties

Holding to truths
Spiritual issues
Externally based stress
General sadness
Processing loss issues
Past heartache
Letting go of trauma
Creative issues
Emotional resilience
Relationship issues
Sexual fears
Control of others
Intimacy issues
Fear of Ming

FIGURE 1.7: INTERNAL PATHOGENIC BODY REGIONS

THE PATH TO DAO

Was good health the main aim of Daoism? Yes and no. Of course nobody wants to live in a state of discomfort or disease but gaining good health was only the foundational stage of Daoist practices, even practices from within the medical tradition. The beginning states of spiritual practice and attaining good health are one and the same in Daoism, as it is through the good health and harmonious interaction of the three bodies of man that the road to Dao becomes apparent. Figure 1.8 illustrates this concept.

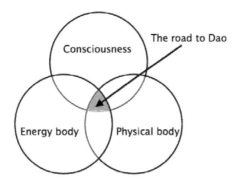

FIGURE 1.8: THE ROAD TO DAO

At the centre point, which is found when the three bodies of man are harmonised, is the entrance to the Xuan Men – the Mysterious Pass. It is through here that the states of stillness can be found which lead a practitioner through the various layers of spiritual cultivation. Opening this gateway was the aim of the Daoist schools and good health was the foundation through which this gateway was opened. Good health was the first stage, not the final goal.

Whilst Dao Yin exercises are highly unlikely to lead you all the way to the state of being able to open and access the Mysterious Pass, they are a useful tool for building the foundational stages of good and vibrant health, both physical and emotional.

CHAPTER 2

THE JING BODY

The energetic pathways of the meridian system are well documented in the Daoist tradition. Chinese medicine textbooks and many Qi Gong texts outline the nature of the meridians, as well as their functions and their relationship to deeper elements of the energy body such as the three Dan Tien. Due to the amount of written material on the aspect of the human body that exists in the realm of Qi there is often a mistaken belief that the ancient Daoists completely ignored the physical body in their teachings. This is far from the truth. The skin, muscles, bones and connective tissues of our physical structure make up the vehicle that contains the meridian system and its associated energetic elements. In this book all aspects of the physical body will be referred to collectively as the Jing body.

The Jing body is actually one step down from our essential essence; it is the condensed result of the transformational process of consciousness moving into the realm of existence. In this way, as spirit enters the realm of Heaven and Earth it slows down and manifests as a body – a vehicle through which to experience life and interact with the rest of the physical world. This physical body consists of the cells, tissues, fluids, bones, muscles, etc., that are studied and understood in Western biological sciences. The Qi and spirit of man resides and interacts with this physical body to create the changing processes which we move through over the course of our lives.

Two aspects of the physical body which are particularly important for Dao Yin training and indeed all of the Daoist arts are the Pi Fu and Jing Jin systems. These two systems of the body are rarely described in much detail in internal arts manuals, and are really only given a vague nod in the majority of Chinese medicine practices. This is a shame, as understanding and utilising these two systems in internal arts practices leads to higher levels of physical ability and improved health.

It is a great mistake to dedicate yourself solely to the study of the internal arts and completely neglect the physical body; to work in this way is unbalanced. The quality of a person's Qi may be as smooth and as healthy as can be, but if the vehicle transporting it, the physical body, is in a poor state then all their training will amount to very little. The legend of Bodhidharma entering the Shaolin monastery and teaching the monks forms of physical exercise which would go on to become Shaolin Gong Fu demonstrates this point very well. Whether or not the legend is true, it shows how the monks had to add another practice to their daily regime in order to look after their physical bodies, which were becoming weak from the prolonged sitting practice they were undertaking.

What follows is a discussion of the various elements of the Jing body which are important in the study of Dao Yin exercises; namely the Pi Fu system and the Jing Jin system.

PI FU

The Pi Fu system is essentially the body's skin. It surrounds the entire body and exists as the outermost layer of the physical body; thus it is the external barrier between our inner body and the external environment. It houses the body hair, contains the pores of the skin which enable, amongst other things, the movement of the Qi field, and provides a root for the Wei Qi, a protective energetic layer that guards us against which protects us from invading pathogens and emotional information. In order to understand these functions of the Pi Fu system we need first to understand the basic structure of the body's skin (Figure 2.1).

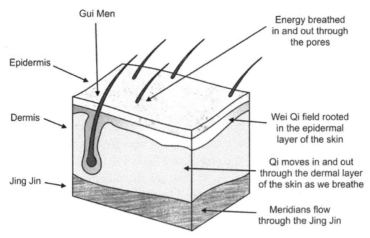

FIGURE 2.1: THE PI FU AND THE UNDERLYING JING JIN

The most Yang layer of the Pi Fu system corresponds to the epidermal layer of the skin. This is the layer within which the root of the Wei Qi field flows. This is the layer of Qi which is known in English as the 'Guardian Qi' field. The strength of this protective layer of Qi determines how well we fight off external disease which would otherwise invade deeper into the body, leading to the development of sickness. This layer of Qi is a combination of Qi that we draw from the food we eat, along with our original essence; the strength of these two combined governs the strength of our Wei Qi field. Further layers of the Wei Qi field permeate out from the root of the Wei Qi field, through our emotional defensive layer and out into our spiritual layers, which defend us from more ethereal energies that would otherwise negatively affect us.

The epidermal layer of the Pi Fu system also includes the countless Gui Men which are said to sit in the hair follicles and sweat glands of the body. Gui Men can be translated as 'Ghost Gates' and refers to the locations where Qi moves in and out of the body through the expansion and contraction of our auric Qi field as we breathe. The breathing controls the movement of this Qi field as shown in Figure 2.2.

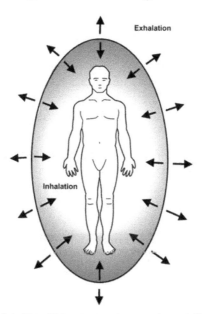

FIGURE 2.2: THE MOVEMENT OF THE AURIC QI FIELD

The movement of the Qi through the Gui Men enables the body to absorb informational Qi vibrations from the external environment. If our health and connection to nature are balanced, then this is a great course of acquired Qi, but if we are out of balance or our filtering Wei Qi system is weak then we will draw in toxins from the environment through these gates. In shamanic Daoist sects these pathogenic energies were thought to be ghosts – hence the term 'Gui Men'. In medical Daoist practices these pathogens are simply identified as forms of Qi and generally labelled as the pathogenic factors of Wind-Heat, Wind-Cold, Damp, Cold, Heat and Dryness. Within the Traditional Chinese Medicine (TCM) tradition this list of pathogens became Wind, Heat, Cold, Damp, Dryness and Summer-Heat. Different traditions will have slightly different understandings.

Penetrating the three layers of the Pi Fu system, down through the Jing Jin layer into the meridians, are the major gateways of Qi which we know as meridian points. These portals of information enable strong movements of Qi in and out of the body; these are points utilised in therapeutic treatments such as acupuncture.

The different areas of the Pi Fu system are labelled according to the meridian pathways that run beneath them. The locations of the Pi Fu zones are shown in Figure 2.3.

A therapist of the Daoist tradition will use visible and tangible signs such as textures, lumps and colours in these different areas to identify imbalances in the Qi of the meridians that correspond to these areas. This is because the stagnant information from the meridians will naturally want to be expelled from the body via the Gui Men and this process leaves marks of imbalance upon the skin.

If the Pi Fu system is free from imbalance then there will be no 'binding' of the skin layers and there will be no obvious marks from pathogens travelling along the various meridians beneath the Pi Fu system. As you practise Dao Yin exercises or similar movements your skin should slide to some degree over the tissues below. The more you practise, the more this will begin to happen to your skin, and after some time you will begin to feel the connected, elasticated nature of the skin like a giant bag encasing your whole body. You will feel as though you are 'vacuum packed' in your skin!

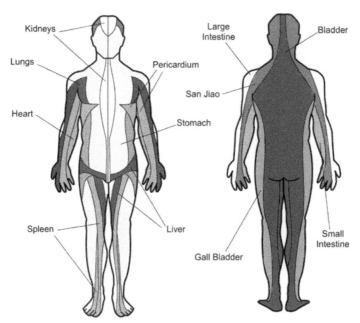

FIGURE 2.3: THE PI FU ZONES

JING JIN

Arguably the most important aspect of the body for the practice of Dao Yin exercises is the Jing Jin system. This is the layer of muscles, connective tissue and fascia beneath the Pi Fu system, which acts as a kind of physical 'riverbed' for the Qi of the meridian system as it travels through the body. Jing Jin can be translated as 'tendon pathways', although the term Jin ('tendons') actually refers to the muscles, tendons, ligaments and connective tissue which run along the lines of these physical pathways. They are a vitally important part of the knowledge base for the internal arts, as they imply a degree of connection that is not generally dealt with in the study of the muscular system in Western Sciences. In Western biology, muscles and their related tendons are generally studied independently of each other. They are seen as little more than a contracting piece of tissue which enables the levers of the bones to move; there is little in the way of understanding how these muscles form one connected system. Fortunately this is beginning to change as several pioneering authors and manual therapists such as Meyers

(2008)[1] begin to challenge this view through their study of the myofascial network of the body, which is essentially the Jing Jin system that has been part of the Daoist knowledge base for centuries.

The pathways of the Jing Jin follow the line of the meridian pathways and are generally labelled as such. For example, the Heart Jing Jin is named after the Heart meridian which runs along the same pathway. Despite these names there is no direct connection between the organs and the Jing Jin; communication instead takes place between the organs and the Jing Jin via the intermediary of the meridian system.

Following is a brief discussion of the pathways of the 12 key Jing Jin. Labels are given with regard to the individual muscles that make up the Jing Jin, but also included, of course, are the ligaments, tendons and fascia pathways that run along these lines. Muscle names are included for ease of reference. Note that classically the Jing Jin are always described as moving from the extremities inwards towards the core of the body. Although they actually encourage Qi flow in both directions along each meridian, I have remained true to the classical directions of flow when describing each Jing Jin pathway. The outlined and shaded area then shows each Jing Jin pathway. (This is really too literal a way of showing the layout of the connective tissues, as they actually spread out into the rest of the body like a kind of 'connective tissue cobweb' – but it is adequate for the purpose of illustrating which areas of the body are involved in each Jing Jin.) Note also that the Jing Jin pathways do not follow the same route through the body as the Pi Fu zones.

1   Meyers, T. (2008) *Anatomy Trains: Myofascial Meridians for Manual and Movement Therapists*, 2nd edn. London: Churchill Livingstone, Elsevier.

Heart Jing Jin

The Heart Jing Jin originates at the radial corner of the little finger; it travels to the wrist and then ascends along the medial aspect of the arm, via the elbow to the axilla. Here it conjoins with the Lung Jing Jin and descends via an internal connection through the diaphragm all the way down to the umbilicus. Key muscles included in the pathway of the Heart Jing Jin include the *abductor digiti minimi*, the *flexor digitorum superficialis*, the brachialis tendon and part of *pectoralis major*. Figure 2.4 shows the pathway and inclusive muscles of the Heart Jing Jin. All channels are bilateral on the body.

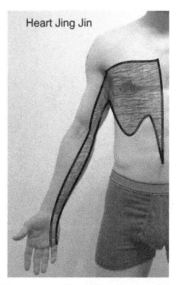

FIGURE 2.4: THE HEART JING JIN

Physical imbalances include pain and tension anywhere along the line of the Jing Jin, as well as cramping sensations in the diaphragm and upper abdomen.

Small Intestine Jing Jin

The Small Intestine Jing Jin originates at the tip of the little finger and ascends the arm to the medial aspect of the elbow. It then continues upwards along the length of the arm to connect with the scapula. This pathway then travels up the neck, around the ear and across the cheek to terminate in the temple area. Key muscles included in the Small Intestine Jing Jin are *extensor carpi ulnaris*, the *triceps*, the middle *deltoid*, *infraspinatus*, the upper *trapezius*, the *masseter* muscles and the *temporalis* muscles. Figure 2.5 shows the pathway of the Small Intestine Jing Jin.

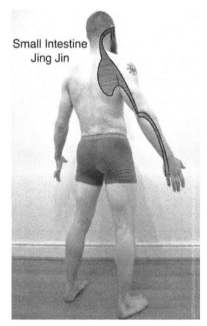

FIGURE 2.5: THE SMALL INTESTINE JING JIN

Imbalances of the Small Intestine Jing Jin manifest as pain and spasms in the little finger, pain and tightness anywhere along the length of the Jing Jin, and earache that feels as if it is 'swelling'.

Pericardium Jing Jin

The Pericardium Jing Jin originates on the palmar aspect (on the underside) of the middle finger and then ascends along the middle of the inner arm via the elbow to the axilla. It then spreads across the chest region, whilst an internal branch enters the body and terminates in the area of the heart. Key muscles included in the pathway of the Pericardium Jing Jin include the *flexor digitorum superficialis* tendons, *palmaris longus*, *flexor carpi radialis* and *biceps brachialis*. Figure 2.6 shows the pathway and inclusive muscles of the Pericardium Jing Jin.

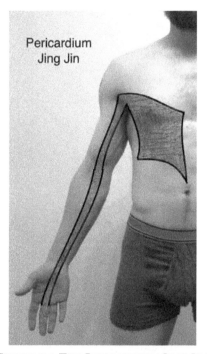

FIGURE 2.6: THE PERICARDIUM JING JIN

Physical imbalances of the Pericardium Jing Jin include pain and spasm of the middle finger, pain and tightness anywhere along the length of the Jing Jin, and cramping sensations of the chest.

San Jiao Jing Jin

The San Jiao Jing Jin originates at the end of the ring finger. From here it ascends the arm to connect at the olecranon of the elbow; it then ascends along the upper arm and crosses the shoulder and neck, ascending past the temple and outer canthus of the eye to connect at the ear. A branch running from the jaw moves internally to connect with the root of the tongue. Key muscles included in the pathway of the San Jiao Jing Jin include *extensor digitorum, brachialis*, the middle *deltoid, platysma* and the *masseter* muscles. Figure 2.7 shows the pathway of the San Jiao Jing Jin.

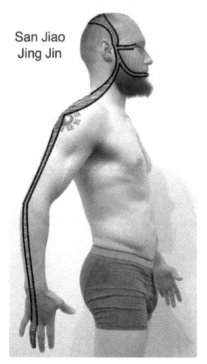

San Jiao
Jing Jin

FIGURE 2.7: THE SAN JIAO JING JIN

Imbalances of the San Jiao Jing Jin include tightness and pain of the ring finger, discomfort along the length of the Jing Jin, or cramping sensations in the base of the tongue.

Spleen Jing Jin

The Spleen Jing Jin originates at the medial side of the big toe. From here it ascends to the medial malleolus and then up to the medial epicondyle of the tibia. It travels upwards along the medial aspect of the thigh to the hip. From here it travels across to the external genitalia before ascending the lower abdomen to the umbilicus. From here it moves internally before spreading through the inside of the ribcage, and then connects to the thoracic area of the spine. Key muscles included in the pathway of the Spleen Jing Jin are *extensor hallucis longus, flexor digitorum longus,* the *soleus* muscles, and *rectus abdominis.* Figure 2.8 shows the pathway and inclusive muscles of the Spleen Jing Jin.

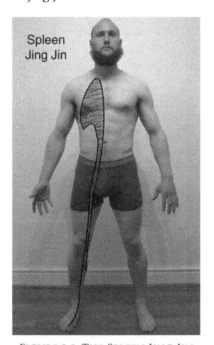

FIGURE 2.8: THE SPLEEN JING JIN

Imbalances along the length of the Spleen Jing Jin include pain and discomfort of the big toe, pain anywhere along the line of the Jing Jin, tenderness along the medial border of the tibia, difficulty rotating the hip joint outwards (it may click as you move) and abdominal cramping.

Stomach Jing Jin

The Stomach Jing Jin originates at the ends of the second and third toes and then travels along the dorsum of the foot to the anterior aspect of the ankle. From here it ascends the anterior of the lower leg to the base of the knee, where it divides into two branches. The first branch travels from the lateral aspect of the knee along the thigh to the hip, wraps around the side of the abdomen and ascends to the lower thoracic region of the back. The second branch ascends the anterior of the thigh and then travels upwards over the abdomen to the supraclavicular fossa. From here it ascends the neck, enwraps the mouth and then continues upwards to surround the eye. A divergent aspect from the neck travels along the jaw, in front of the ear and up to the corner of the temple. Key muscles included in the pathway of the Stomach Jing Jin are *extensor digitorum longus*, *tibialis anterior*, *vastus medialis*, *adductor longus*, *vastus lateralis*, the external obliques, *latissimus dorsi*, *rectus abdominis*, *pectoralis major*, the *platysma*, the *masseter*, *orbicularis oculi*, and *levator labii superioris*. Figure 2.9 shows the pathway and inclusive muscles of the Stomach Jing Jin.

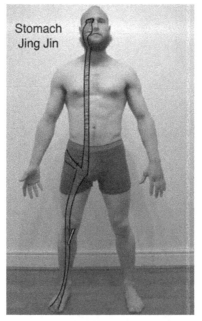

Stomach
Jing Jin

FIGURE 2.9: THE STOMACH JING JIN

Imbalance of the Stomach Jing Jin includes pain and cramping of the second and third toe, tightness anywhere along the length of the Jing Jin, hernia and Wind type (Chinese medical diagnosis) spasms of the eye muscles.

Lung Jing Jin

The Lung Jin Jin originates at the tip of the thumb. It ascends laterally along the forearm to the elbow and continues along the upper arm to the anterior of the shoulder joint. One branch then ascends along the line of the clavicle whilst another descends internally to connect and spread along the surface of the diaphragm. Key muscles included in the pathway of the Lung Jing Jin are *abductor pollicis brevis, brachioradialis, biceps brachii,* the anterior *deltoid* and *subclavius.* Figure 2.10 shows the pathway of the Lung Jing Jin.

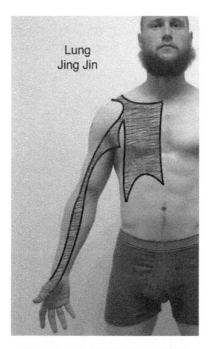

FIGURE 2.10: THE LUNG JIN JIN

Physical imbalances include pain and spasm in the thumb, tightness and discomfort anywhere along the length of the Jing Jin and constriction of the diaphragm, which may, in turn, affect the breathing.

Large Intestine Jing Jin

The Large Intestine Jing Jin originates at the tip of the index finger and thumb. From here it ascends along the forearm to the medial aspect of the elbow. It then travels to the lower border of the shoulder, where it branches into two parts. The first branch spreads across the shoulder blade to connect with the spine. The second branch ascends the neck and travels across the face to the corner of the nose. This branch continues up over the head to connect with the Large Intestine Jing Jin of the opposite side of the body. Key muscles included along the pathway of the Large Intestine Jing Jin are the *extensor digitorum, biceps brachii*, the middle anterior *deltoid,* the *trapezius,* the *platysma, masseter* and *temporalis* muscles. Figure 2.11 shows the pathways and inclusive muscles of the Large Intestine Jing Jin.

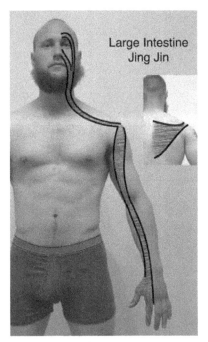

FIGURE 2.11: THE LARGE INTESTINE JING JIN

Physical imbalances along the length of the Large Intestine Jing Jin include pain and spasm in the index finger, pain and tightness along the length of the Jing Jin, the condition known in the West as 'frozen shoulder' and difficulty in looking from side to side.

Kidney Jing Jin

The Kidney Jing Jin originates on the underside of the little toe and travels across the base of the foot along to the heel and medial malleolus. It then travels upwards to the medial epicondyle of the tibia below the knee. From here it ascends the inner thigh to conclude externally at the genitalia. An internal branch ascends up both sides of the spine into the internal occipital region. Key muscles included in the pathway of the Kidney Jing Jin are *flexor digiti minimi brevis*, the plantar fascia, the *gastrocnemius* muscle and *gracilis*. Figure 2.12 shows the pathway of the Kidney Jing Jin.

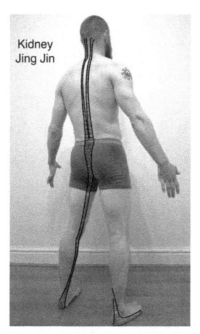

FIGURE 2.12: THE KIDNEY JING JIN

Physical imbalances include pain along the length of the Jing Jin, plantar fasciitis, stiffness when bending and general weakness of the spine and neck.

Bladder Jing Jin

The Bladder Jing Jin originates on the little toe and ascends to the base of the lateral aspect of the knee and the posterior aspect of the calves. From here it travels up the posterior of the thigh and over the buttocks, then ascends parallel to the spine, and divides at the upper medial corner of the scapula. The first branch travels over the scapula to enwrap the thorax before moving round the neck to the edge of the nose. The second branch continues up past the occipital region and over the head. From here it continues until it meets the first branch of the Bladder Jing Jin on the nose. A small branch encompasses the muscles of the upper eye. Key muscles included in the pathway of the Bladder Jing Jin are the extensor tendons, *peroneus longus*, the *gastrocnemius*, the muscles of the popliteal fossa, *biceps femoris*, *semitendinosus*, the gluteal muscles, the *erector spinae*, *latissimus dorsi*, *infraspinatus*, *occipitofrontalis*, *frontalis*, the *platysma*, *sternocleidomastoid*, *pectoralis major* and *serratus anterior*. Figure 2.13 shows the pathway of the Bladder Jing Jin.

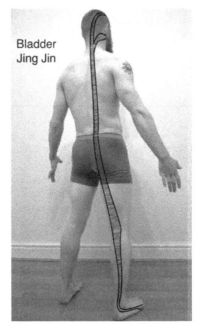

Bladder
Jing Jin

FIGURE 2.13: THE BLADDER JING JIN

Imbalances along the length of the Bladder Jing Jin include tightness and pain, especially along the length of the back. General achiness in the shoulder and area of the clavicle are also signs of possible imbalance in this Jing Jin.

Liver Jing Jin

The Liver Jing Jin originates on the dorsum of the big toe. It ascends the foot to the medial malleolus, then travels along the leg to the medial side of the knee and upwards to the groin area, where it terminates. Key muscles included along the length of the Liver Jing Jin are the *soleus* muscles, *vastus medialis, pectineus* and the base of the *rectus abdominis* muscles. Figure 2.14 shows the pathway of the Liver Jing Jin.

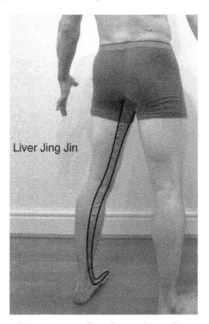

Liver Jing Jin

FIGURE 2.14: THE LIVER JING JIN

Imbalances along the length of the Liver Jing Jin include pain and tightness, cramping of the big toe, or even a feeling of tightness and cramping at the base of the genitalia in men.

Gall Bladder Jing Jin

The Gall Bladder Jing Jin originates at the lateral edge of the fourth toe, and travels to the lateral malleolus. From here it ascends the lateral aspect of the leg and up to the hip, where it divides into three branches below the line of the lower hips. The first branch travels across the buttocks to connect internally with the sacrum. The second branch continues across the lateral aspect of the abdomen to the neck, where it continues over the head to connect with the Gall Bladder Jing Jin of the opposite side of the body. The third branch travels around the front of the leg to connect into the inner thigh. A divergent branch from the area of the ear travels around the face to connect with the muscles of the lower eye. Key muscles of the Gall Bladder Jing Jin include *extensor digitorum longus, tibialis anterior, tensor fasciae latae, gluteus maximus*, the external obliques, *serratus anterior, pectoralis major, masseater, sternocleinomastoid, temporalis* and *levator labii superioris*. Figure 2.15 shows the pathway of the Gall Bladder Jing Jin.

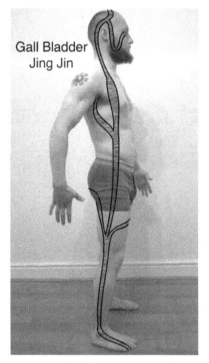

FIGURE 2.15: THE GALL BLADDER JING JIN

Imbalances in the length of the Gall Bladder Jing Jin include pain anywhere along the length of the Jing Jin. Pain of the outer knee and lateral aspect of the abdomen are common, along with facial twitches and a feeling of 'stuck-ness' in the side of the head, just above the ears.

THE PATHWAYS OF CONNECTION

What is most important about the pathways of the Jing Jin is that these are the key pathways of physical integration along the body. Do not think of the muscles of the Jing Jin as isolated parts; they are part of one continuous chain of connected muscles, tissues and fascia which, if healthy, feel much like a long line of elastic when they are stretched. It is along the integrated lengths of the Jing Jin that we move, stretch and twist during practices such as Dao Yin. This helps to deliver information more efficiently along the length of the associated meridians, as well as ensuring a higher level of core stability and power.

If the Jing Jin are relaxed, correctly conditioned and free from stagnation then you will get a sense of true connection along each line, but if there is imbalance present then instead you will experience the individual parts of the Jing Jin moving each in isolation from the next part. Each muscle will appear to move on its own; to the trained eye it is easy to tell the level of skill of an internal artist by observing the degree of connection they possess along the lines of the Jing Jin.

I often explain to my students that they are attempting to connect the various elements of the Jing Jin system into one integrated whole so that it feels as if they are wearing a kind of biological wetsuit when they move. This elasticated feeling should be present over the entire body. There are several factors involved in the health of the Jing Jin, which govern whether or not it is possible to connect along their lengths. These are as follows:

- The Jing Jin must not be held in tension. Tension causes the different areas of the Jing Jin to contract and separate from each other. Tension leads to isolation of body parts and disconnected movement.

- The Jing Jin must not be too slack. If the Jing Jin are too slack then information cannot be transferred along their length, and so disconnection occurs. Slackness in the Jing Jin usually occurs as a result of either bad posture or a poor diet that is weakening the Spleen, which energetically governs the health of the Jing Jin. There must be a good balance between not being too slack or too tense; this is often the most problematic area when beginners start working with the Jing Jin.

- The Jing Jin must be lengthened through stretching. If a person is not flexible enough and there is limited mobility in the joints of the body, then the Jing Jin will not be sufficiently lengthened and information cannot be transferred through them.

- The health of the meridian associated with the Jing Jin must be balanced, free-flowing and free of stagnation, as any problems in this respect will manifest physically in the Jing Jin, resulting in disconnection.

- Physical injuries sustained along the length of the Jing Jin will contribute to their tightening, which leads to disconnection. They must be minimised and worked on through gentle mobilising and stretching exercises. It is possible to condition the Jing Jin to compensate and 'work around' the vast majority of musculo-skeletal injuries which sit along the length of the Jing Jin.

- Any movement utilising the Jing Jin successfully will incorporate a twisting, opening or lengthening movement along the length of the whole Jing Jin. The joints and muscles of the entire Jing Jin will all be manipulated at the same time; it is partly for this reason that so much importance is attributed to hand positions within the internal arts. The fingers act as the origin of half of the Jing Jin, and help to lengthen them fully out.

Exercises such as the Dragon Dao Yins contained in this book enable us to condition the Jing Jin so that they connect together successfully. These principles are then easy to apply to all other Daoist internal arts, and indeed other movement arts. I had the opportunity to teach a ballet group in the UK for a while. I taught them the movements of the Dragon Dao Yins and helped them to connect along the length of the Jing Jin; after a few weeks of training they all said that they had a higher degree of bodily connection which carried across into their dancing.

Gaining a Sense of Connection

Here is an easy exercise which will show you how connected your Jing Jin pathways currently are. If they are already pretty well lengthened and connected, then when you perform the exercise you will get a strong sense of movement along the entire length of the Jing Jin; it will feel as though your muscles are sliding in one connected line beneath the level of your skin. If your Jing Jin are disconnected, then you will either feel nothing or you will feel movement isolated in the area of your forearm.

Sit in a chair or with legs folded. As an alternative, you can also do this exercise standing. Extend up the top of your head and lengthen your spine so that you are sitting upright. Relax your shoulders and ensure that they are not raised. Extend your right arm as shown in Figure 2.16.

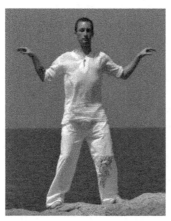

FIGURE 2.16: BEGINNING THE CONNECTION EXERCISE

Ensure that your elbow is bent as shown in Figure 2.16 and dropped straight down towards the floor. Now slightly extend the arm very slowly and bring the hand into the 'hook position' shown in Figure 2.17. (This hand position will be familiar to most practitioners of Taijiquan.) Co-ordinate the movement with your breathing and slowly move between the two positions.

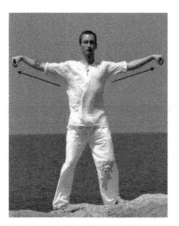

FIGURE 2.17: THE HOOK POSITION

As you close the fingers into the hook position you should gently stretch the back of the hand and lengthen the fingers as if the hand position is forming around a ball. This enables the Jing Jin on the back of the hand to connect together.

Perform this exercise for a few minutes and try to 'tune in' to what is happening elsewhere in your body. If you have successfully connected the Jing Jin together then you should feel movement elsewhere in the body. Essentially this movement should lengthen along the Small Intestine, Large Intestine and San Jiao Jing Jin pathways as you form the hook position. This means that you should feel deep movement along the line of these pathways along the arm, as well as movement of the fascia and muscles around the area of the clavicle and across the side of the neck and face. Those with a great deal of internal awareness and connection will also be able to feel movement deep inside the body around the area of the diaphragm but it is uncommon to feel this in the early stages of learning this exercise.

If you cannot feel this movement then try adjusting the movement a little; change your posture slightly to ensure that no part of the Jing Jin will be too slack and consequently disconnected. Of course, you must also relax and lengthen everything as well.

If you can feel the movement, then well done; this is essentially the movement and connection principle which is practised throughout all of the Dragon Dao Yin exercises, although the complexity of the movements enables these movements to take place over the entire body.

FUNCTIONS OF THE JING JIN SYSTEM

The Jing Jin system encompasses the entire body and performs several important functions. These include bodily connection as discussed above, as well as the transference of mechanical and energetic information in and out of the body and, most important of all, providing a strong vessel for the meridians to flow through. There are many crossovers between the Jing Jin system and the network of fascia (Jin Mo in Chinese), which are currently being explored by more pioneering manual therapists and anatomists.

Transference of Information

In order to understand the passing of information into and out of the body via the Jing Jin system, we must first understand the comparative depths of various components of the human body system. There is a sequential order of layers through which information passes from the external environment to our inner universe and vice versa. These layers are shown in Figure 2.18.

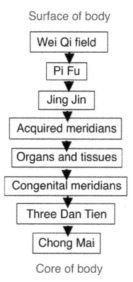

FIGURE 2.18: THE LAYERS OF THE HUMAN BODY SYSTEM

This is a simplified model of the layers of the body; there are other elements not shown in the diagram, but this level of knowledge is adequate for working with Dao Yin practices. It shows us how information from the environment has to pass through the protecting filter of the external Wei Qi field before it reaches the Pi Fu layer of our skin. From here information enters the Gui Men (part of the Pi Fu system) and then continues on to the Jing Jin which contains the energetic pathways of the acquired meridians. This information is then carried from the acquired meridians into the organs and tissues of the body as well as the congenital meridians. The deeper levels consist of the Dan Tien and the central branch of the Chong Mai, which marks the energetic core of our body. Note though that it is highly unlikely for energetic pathogens to reach any deeper than the layer of the organs and tissues.

In the opposite direction we transfer Qi back out from our inner universe into the external environment. This is the nature of our symbiotic relationship with the world in which we live. We are the world and the world is us. Much of this Qi is pure vibrational energy developed from our innate consciousness, but along with this travels toxic energetic information which the body will want to expel back out of the body via the Gui Men and selected meridian points. Dao Yin exercises are essentially designed to heighten this process and make it more efficient.

We want this information transference process to take place as smoothly as possible. To ensure that this happens we fully activate the energy system through internal practices such as Nei Gong and Qi Gong; we apply the health-governing principles of Yang Sheng Fa to our lifestyles to help protect our Jing, boost our Wei Qi and strengthen our energy body; and finally we condition the Jing Jin. The layers of the Jing Jin are a key component in this transference of information, as they enable vibrational information to pass through if they are in good condition. The key to this is treating the Jing Jin as if it were the 'skin of a drum'. When a drum is being struck the skin vibrates and this, in conjunction with a hollow space, produces an audible sound which is essentially just a vibration. If the skin of the drum was slack then there would be no vibration, the power of the strike to the drum skin would be absorbed and no information would be passed through the skin. If the drum skin is too tight then there can be no vibration, no information travels through the skin into the hollow space and no sound is produced. This is exactly how the Jing Jin works; we must find this harmonious balance between too slack and too tight (tense) so that the vibration (Qi) can pass both into and out of the body.

This information which is passed through these layers takes two forms. The first is Qi, vibrational information which governs our health and level of connection to the environment. The second is mechanical/sensory information such as pressure, temperature, etc. This information passes directly from the outside world into the inner universe of our body via the Jing Jin. This shows us the potential therapeutic value of touch; a tender caress from a loved one delivers positive information down into the body, whilst a rough blow has the opposite effect. It is the Jing Jin that delivers the information from therapies such as massage into the body, and it is the skill of the massage therapist that dictates how healthy this information is; too rough, with little care, and a massage can be extremely damaging to the energetic matrix of the body. As a simple rule, if you feel energetically low, physically drained or emotionally down after a massage then the wrong information has been transferred into the body. An exception to this is medical massage, which can produce what is known as a 'healing crisis', and it is important to be able to distinguish between the two in order to ascertain whether or not a particular therapy or therapist is good for you.

A VESSEL FOR THE MERIDIANS

The acquired meridians of the body are situated deeper in the body than the Jing Jin pathways, as can be seen in Figure 2.18. This is because the meridians actually flow through the Jing Jin; they are contained in them. The health of the Jing Jin dictates just how efficiently the flow of Qi information along the line of the meridians takes place. Quite simply, tightness in the Jing Jin will lead to blockages in the meridian, which in turn will lead to stagnation, the main cause of disease. Too slack Jing Jin through bad posture or an unhealthy lack of stretching and conditioning in a person's life can weaken the vessel through which the meridian travels; the result is a dispersal of Qi, which leads to energetic deficiency. This underlines the importance of Jing Jin work for general health as well as development of arts such as Nei Gong, meditation and internal martial arts which rely upon the flow of Qi in the meridian system.

CORE POWER

An interesting aspect of work with the Jing Jin is the increase in physical power that comes as a result of the training. As the Jing Jin start to connect together they begin to assist in developing power which comes from the core of the body. Rather than using isolated muscles when moving, lifting, and so on, you begin to use the entire body via the Jing Jin system and the mechanical information which is passed along its length. This is much healthier for a person, as it means that any work carried out over the course of a person's life relies on force distributed throughout the whole of the body, rather than originating in isolated muscle groups.

For practitioners of martial arts this has obvious benefits and it is the Jing Jin on which the majority of internal styles are based. My opinion is different from that of many other teachers, who place a great deal of importance on transferring Qi through the meridians system when teaching arts such as Taijiquan, Baguazhang and Xingyiquan; instead I place more emphasis on the use of the Jing Jin until higher levels of training are reached. The level of connection attained through this style of training is much greater and Fa Jin power is much higher. The Dragon Dao Yin exercises are excellent exercises to help condition and work with the Jing Jin in preparation for, or as an adjunct to, martial arts training. The principles learnt here are easy to transfer across to the internal martial arts.

DAO YIN AND JING JIN

As well as using breath work, mental intention and directed Qi flow, Dao Yin exercises lengthen the Jing Jin, which are twisted and stretched by the various postures and movements. Figure 2.19 shows how two different postures taken from the Dragon Dao Yin utilise the Jing Jin.

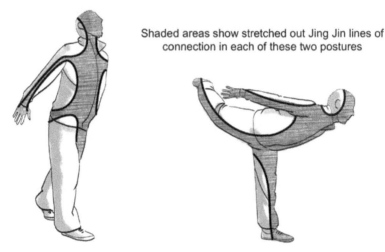

Shaded areas show stretched out Jing Jin lines of connection in each of these two postures

FIGURE 2.19: DRAGON DAO YIN AND JING JIN

Whilst Dao Yin movements are easy to learn, the real skill comes from learning how to connect along the length of each Jing Jin during the movements. Lengthening must take place simultaneously along the entire length of the Jing Jin to encourage a healthy transference of information, core connection and efficient Qi flow through the associated meridian. Remember that you should be striving to attain that feeling of wearing a biological 'wetsuit' throughout your practice.

THE GIRDLING MERIDIAN

An extra meridian which is involved in connection along the lines of the Jing Jin is the girdling meridian. This meridian is part of the congenital aspect of the energy body and unique in that it is the only meridian which travels horizontally through the body. It enwraps the lower abdomen like a belt. Energetically its role is primarily to govern the rotation of the lower Dan Tien by working as a kind of energetic gyroscope. It also has extending branches which energetically enwrap the rest of the meridian system. For more information on the congenital energy system please refer to my previous book, *Daoist Nei Gong: The Philosophical Art of Change.*

Figure 2.20 shows the girdling meridian. The associated key muscles are the internal obliques, as well as the deeper psoas muscles, which are also involved in the girdling meridian Jing Jin.

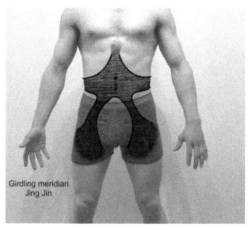

Girdling meridian
Jing Jin

FIGURE 2.20: THE GIRDLING MERIDIAN

Within Dao Yin practice it is the girdling meridian's Jing Jin that connects across the body. In general the 12 key Jing Jin transfer force vertically through the body along their length. If, however, the force is transferred from one side of the body to the other, as in the posture shown in Figure 2.21, then it has to pass through the girdling meridian Jing Jin. As you can see, this is generally achieved through postures which involve twisting the torso. This would obviously apply to many of the Dragon Dao Yin movements as well as the internal martial art of Baguazhang.

At first the twisting movements in Dao Yin training help to condition and connect the force across the body. With time the twist is no longer required; as the Jing Jin of the girdling meridian becomes more adept, it automatically begins to integrate all of the Jing Jin into one unified whole which is mirrored across the body; at this stage all power becomes concentrated in the core of the body.

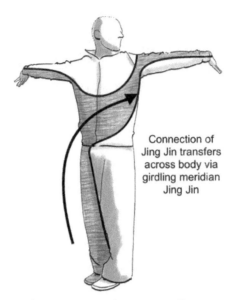

Connection of
Jing Jin transfers
across body via
girdling meridian
Jing Jin

FIGURE 2.21: TRANSFERRING ALONG THE GIRDLING JING JIN

UNDERSTANDING THE JING JIN

In order to fully understand the Jing Jin and their impact upon your training it is worth spending some time getting to know their pathways. I would recommend re-reading this chapter a few times and familiarising yourself with the pathways of the various Jing Jin; this will help with developing a good feeling and understanding of the Dragon Dao Yin exercises. Try stretching your body in different ways along the lines of the Jing Jin; play with various movements you may know from your own practices, such as Qi Gong, Taijiquan or yoga, and try to link them to the various Jing Jin; this will help you to develop a tangible, experiential understanding of these lines of connection.

CHAPTER 3

THE NATURE OF PATHOGENS

The key role of Dao Yin exercises is to purge imbalances from the body. These imbalances take the form of pathogenic Qi which travels through the meridian system causing stagnation and disease. This pathogenic information comes from two main sources: from the external environment and from within us, mainly by way of our emotions. Whatever the source of the imbalance, the result is pathogenic Qi, often known as Xie Qi, which we need to clear from the body. Pathogenic Qi left in the energetic system will gradually lead to stagnation of energetic flow in this area of the body, as well as serving as the root for physical disease, psychological imbalance or both. The root of any physical disease has to lie in the energetic realm, according to Daoism, and often it goes deeper than this, having its root in the mind and the emotions. Clearing this Qi from the body will break the root of the disease, leading to an improvement in our health.

EXTERNALLY BASED PATHOGENIC INFORMATION

In my previous book, *Heavenly Streams: Meridian Theory in Nei Gong*, I discussed the nature of externally based pathogenic information in great detail, so it will only be covered here in brief to avoid unnecessary reproduction of information.

The Daoist tradition states that human beings live between two great forces, the extreme Yang entity of Heaven and the extreme Yin of Earth. Serving as two great poles, they exert their influence upon us throughout the course of our lives. In classical *Yi Jing* (I Ching) theory, Yang is indicated with a solid line, whilst Yin is indicated with a broken line. If we connect these three points together as show in Figure 3.1, we get the Chinese character Ren, meaning 'person'.

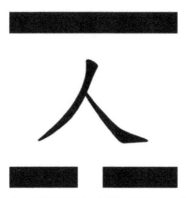

FIGURE 3.1: REN BETWEEN HEAVEN AND EARTH

In the *Yi Jing* or *Classic of Changes* three Yin or Yang lines are combined to form eight spiritual symbols known as trigrams or Gua. These eight symbols represent the interactions of Heaven (Yang) and Earth (Yin), which govern the ebb and flow of Qi of the world we live in. Three Yang lines indicate pure Yang or Heaven. Three Yin lines indicate pure Yin or Earth. These two symbols are known as Qian and Kun. If we are to represent the energetic world symbolically then we can lift Qian to the upper pole and move Kun to the lower pole, with the other six symbols between these two poles as shown in Figure 3.2.

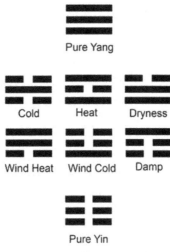

FIGURE 3.2: THE EIGHT GUA

The six symbols that sit between Heaven and Earth show the different ways in which Qi can form as Yin and Yang mix together. These six symbols represent the six key environmental forms of Qi, which exert their influence upon our mind and bodies. They exist in the environment which surrounds us, and at different times of year different Gua energies are dominant. If our relationship to these forms of environmental Qi is balanced then their influence is beneficial, but if it is unbalanced then they can lead to sickness. For example, the Kan Gua, which is shown by two Yin lines surrounding a Yang line, represents the energetic quality of Cold in the environment. During the winter this Gua is dominant, meaning that we can be subjected to extremes of Cold. If we are not internally strong enough to repel this energy then it can invade the body, leading to Cold-based diseases such as influenza, chills or sinus issues. The study of these externally based pathogenic energies is a large part of Chinese medicine and medical Qi Gong.

Any of these pathogens entering the body can lead to imbalance and disease and through practices such as Dao Yin it is possible to help the body expel these pathogens, alleviating symptoms which may be related to them.

INTERNALLY BASED PATHOGENIC DISEASE

Since none of my previous books have discussed the nature of internally based pathogens in any real detail, they will be the subject of most of this chapter. It is important to remember that we are subjected to pathogenic Qi equally from both sources, from outside of the body and from within. Both of these pathogenic sources result in the formation of similar forms of negative Qi, which can be expelled through Dao Yin practice.

Internally based pathogens are produced by the mind, and in particular the emotional experiences that it is subjected to. The human psyche is divided into two main sections: the Xian Tian or 'congenital' aspect and the Hou Tian or the 'acquired' aspect. They represent the movement from a pure, unsullied state of being towards a state distorted by life experiences, biases and triviality. The state of the congenital mind is one of true stillness and comprehension, whilst the acquired mind exists in a constant state of flux and change. The congenital aspect of human consciousness sits at the core of our psyche, surrounded by the layers of the acquired mind which we have built up over the course of our lives. This is shown in Figure 3.3.

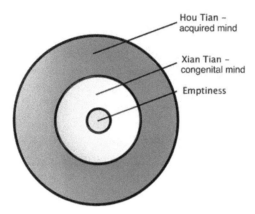

Hou Tian –
acquired mind

Xian Tian –
congenital mind

Emptiness

FIGURE 3.3: THE XIAN TIAN AND THE HOU TIAN SHEN

The congenital consciousness is also known as the 'true self'. It is the part of us that has the potential to access the divine information of the Dao if we are able to access it. Many people never manage to experience connection to their congenital self, instead living out their daily lives from an acquired state of mind. Some people have inadvertent experiences of brief connection to their congenital nature and these short experiences of divine connection can lead to sudden insight or divine understanding. For those who experience this connection it is often life-changing, as they are forced to reconsider everything about their existence. It is the aim of all Daoist practices to lead a practitioner towards direct connection to the congenital self.

The acquired aspect of human consciousness is subject to the movements of the emotions, which move like waves over the ocean of the mind. Each and every thought we have causes disturbances in the maelstrom of emotional energy which is generated by the acquired mind, and over the course of our lives these emotional experiences create our false sense of self; the egocentric concept of self we have which disconnects us from the divine. That being said, the acquired mind is not seen as negative, it is just what it is. The human mind works in this way and this is what we have to work with. Daoism always takes a pragmatic stance on such matters.

The acquired aspect of our consciousness is divided into five key aspects of spirit known as the Hun, the Po, the Yi, the Zhi and the Shen. These five composite parts of our consciousness interact with each other, our inner self and the outside world to create all of the movements and mechanics of psyche which cause us to think, experience and act. In contrast to this the congenital nature is actually only experienced when the five spirits are combined into one unified spiritual entity which gives us access to the true self.

The five spirits each reside in a different physical organ and create a different emotional response when they are out of balance. When in perfect harmony they instead produce a virtuous aspect of nature and these are all listed in Table 3.1.

TABLE 3.1: THE FIVE SPIRITS, EMOTIONS AND VIRTUES

Spirit	Organ of Residence	Emotion	Virtue
Hun	Liver	Anger	Patience
Po	Lungs	Grief	Courage
Yi	Spleen	Worry	Empathy
Zhi	Kidneys	Fear	Wisdom
Shen	Heart	Joy	Contentment

In the vast majority of cases it is the emotions rather than the virtues which we experience on a regular basis. According to Daoist theory all these emotions are nothing more than waves of energy which move through the body in different ways, producing energetic reactions. The subjective experience we have of these movements of energy through the body is an external emotion. Emotions are not seen as negative in the Daoist arts until they reach a point where we become over-attached to them. Once we associate who we are with one of these emotional states and allow this state to become our standpoint for experiencing everything else in life, then we will begin to move further and further out of energetic balance until disease develops.

EMOTIONAL CONNECTION TO THE ORGANS

An interesting aspect of the Daoist arts is that each of the key organs we have in our body governs an emotional aspect of our mind. In Daoism nothing energetic or spiritual can exist without there being a physical entity that anchors it in existence. Conversely, nothing physical can exist without having a root in the spiritual and energetic realms. It is this co-existence of physicality, energy and spirit that forms the basis for the teachings of the entire tradition.

Each of our five spirits is rooted in a key organ of the body as shown in Table 3.1. Each of these spirits dictates a different emotional energy which is given off into the body when we react to particular experiences we may have. Most people have an uneven balance amongst the spirits and organs, which means that they will have more of a tendency towards one or two emotional states, whilst others will be there in the background. The emotions will have a direct effect upon their root organ, i.e. an excess of a particular emotion will begin to cause ill health in the organ it pertains to. For example, excessive, prolonged experiences of anger and frustration will gradually begin to damage the organ of the Liver and its associated elements in the body, according to Chinese medical theory.

Each of the key organs (known as Zang organs) are paired with a secondary organ (known as a Fu organ) which work to try to keep the emotions in balance. The secondary organs in this partnership each dictate a cognitive aspect of psyche which works to keep our emotional experiences in balance and appropriate to our life experiences. The organ pairings are shown in Table 3.2.

TABLE 3.2: PAIRED ORGAN SYSTEMS

Zang Organ	Fu Organ	Zang Emotion	Fu Cognition
Heart	Small Intestine	Joy	Sense of purity
Spleen	Stomach	Worry	Digests ideas
Lungs	Large Intestine	Grief	Enables letting go
Kidneys	Bladder	Fear	Emotional security
Liver	Gall Bladder	Anger	Decision making

In Chinese medical theory, if an emotion is particularly out of balance then it is possible to strengthen the paired organ to try to help with the excess energy being produced. For example, if the Liver is out of balance and excessive anger is damaging the body then a Chinese medical therapist may treat the Liver, but they may also work to nourish the Gall Bladder to help alleviate the symptoms. In the same way it is also common to find many medical Qi Gong exercises which aim not just to treat the key organ (such as the Liver) but often work on the secondary organ as well (in this case the Gall Bladder).

The Heart and Small Intestine Paired System

The Heart governs the emotion of joy and all feelings of excitement that we may have. Whilst joy itself is not such a negative experience, it is fleeting in nature. It is a temporary feeling of pleasantness which is nothing compared to the virtuous aspect of divine contentment which the spirit of the Heart is also able to make available to us. The rule of Yin and Yang would tell us that for every joy we experience there must be some sadness to balance it out, and this rollercoaster of emotional ups and downs gradually takes its toll on the organ of the Heart.

The Heart likes feelings of joy, laughter and merriment. These emotions cause the energetic pulse of the Heart to flare up and expand outwards, which is a nice, warming feeling. What things bring us joy in life will depend very much upon how we were brought up, our first experiences of joy and how they programmed us, as well as the strength of the Small Intestine. In Daoist theory the Small Intestine governs our ability to distinguish right from wrong, the ability to sort the 'pure from the impure'. On a physical level this pertains to the digestive processes that take place in the organ of the small intestine itself, whilst on an emotional level the cognitive function of the Small Intestine ensures that our perceived sources of pleasure are from a pure source. Taking pleasure in the pain of others, misdeeds and even sexually deviant pleasures would be seen as an emotional imbalance between the Heart and the Small Intestine. Figure 3.4 shows the relationship of these two organs.

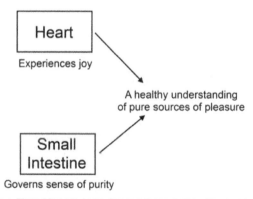

FIGURE 3.4: THE HEART AND SMALL INTESTINE RELATIONSHIP

On an alchemical level it is only possible to connect fully with the spiritual power of the Shen, which resides in the organ of the Heart, once these two organs are emotionally and cognitively in balance with each other. This was one of the key reasons for ethical teachings in classical

Eastern arts; teachings which are too often missing from contemporary Daoist schools.

The Spleen and Stomach Paired System

The Spleen governs our awareness and focus through the action of the spiritual Yi that resides within it. It is also subjected to the emotional experience of worry, along with chronic over-thinking and pensiveness. The majority of these worries are not based in logic and instead are a form of perceived fear projected into the future towards an event which has not yet happened. I have lost count of the amount of times I have had great worries in my life over something I was soon to do, only to find that the actual event held no reason to worry, and none of the various outcomes I had played out over and over in my mind ever came to fruition. This kind of mindset is the emotional reaction of the Spleen when it is out of balance.

The physical organ of the Stomach digests our food and cognitively the Stomach system governs our ability to 'digest ideas'. It is the energy of the Stomach that enables us to take those perceived events described above and mentally 'digest' them. If the Stomach is doing its job efficiently then we should find that with a little consideration none of our worries are founded in anything real, and so the worries should be greatly lessened. Figure 3.5 shows the emotional and cognitive relationship of the Spleen and Stomach.

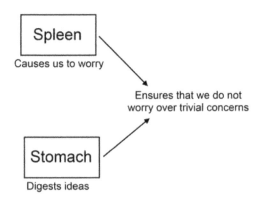

FIGURE 3.5: THE SPLEEN AND STOMACH RELATIONSHIP

The more we can balance the strength of these two organs, the calmer our mind can become; our thoughts settle down and our mental focus becomes stronger. This makes any internal work requiring the Yi much more effective.

The Lungs and Large Intestine Paired System

The Lungs are governed by the spiritual actions of the Po. This is the aspect of our consciousness that is acutely aware of the temporary nature of life. It is the corporeal aspect of self that connects us to the physical world, the false world which is a constant process of breaking down ready for rebirth. This is the organ most affected by sadness and, in particular, grief. This sadness is normally triggered by the loss of something or the perceived fear of the loss of something. It is not necessarily the loss of a loved one, but this would of course be one of the most extreme cases of loss that would affect the emotional energy of the Lungs.

The emotional grief of the Lungs is balanced by the cognitive function of the Large Intestine which governs our ability to 'let go'. On a physical level this is our ability to 'let go' of faecal matter and cognitively it governs our ability to rationalise and let go of things we have lost, whether they be loved ones or possessions. It is the cognitive function of the Large Intestine that also helps us to understand the nature of the finality of life and how this leads to something new: rebirth. Figure 3.6 shows the emotional and cognitive relationship of the Lungs and Large Intestine.

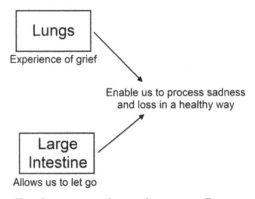

FIGURE 3.6: THE LUNGS AND LARGE INTESTINE RELATIONSHIP

Alchemically it is vitally important that we manage to balance the energy of the Lungs and Large Intestine in order to access the spiritual entity of the Po. This enables us to let go of old sadness and grief which have accumulated within us. It also gives us the divine realisation that death is only part of the great cycle. Note that this realisation has to come from inside, rather than simply from external intellectual teachings, in order to hold any spiritual validity.

The Kidneys and Bladder Paired System

The Kidneys are particularly affected by experiences that generate the emotion of fear within us. These fears can range from phobias and fear of danger through to emotional shocks and trauma, and they cause the Yin and Yang harmonising function of the Kidneys to become damaged, leading to exhaustion and fatigue on the level of our very essence. All of these fears are based on the idea that we are in some kind of danger, and ironically it is this fear itself that actually causes us energetic damage, whether the feared event comes to fruition or not.

The emotional energy of the Kidneys is balanced by the cognitive function of the Bladder, which concerns our level of emotional security. The Bladder meridian is also known as one of the Tai Yang or 'extreme Yang' meridians. It extends along the length of our back and acts as a kind of shield from the energy of the outside world. With regard to invasion from external pathogens it is the Bladder meridian that serves as a 'first point of contact' with these environmental Qi. Emotionally it serves to protect us and this is seen clearly when somebody goes into extreme shock and curls up into a foetal position. They have extended the protective layer of the Bladder meridian around themselves whilst protecting their vulnerable core. Many who are experiencing a lot of emotional fear which the Bladder is trying to keep in check will also find that they naturally want to sleep in this foetal position as well.

The Bladder's cognitive function of controlling our level of emotional security enables us to feel emotionally secure and stand up to the fears that are being projected onto us by the energy coming from the Kidneys. Self-esteem is also connected to the Bladder, and many Bladder issues and weaknesses stem from something that has attacked a person's emotional security or self-esteem. Figure 3.7 shows the emotional and cognitive relationship of the Kidneys and Bladder.

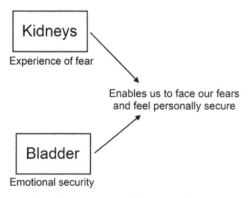

FIGURE 3.7: THE KIDNEYS AND BLADDER RELATIONSHIP

Balancing the energies of the Kidneys and Bladder enables us to understand that there is little to fear. Sense of self becomes irrelevant and since there is no self there is little that can do you harm. This is the foundation understanding upon which true selflessness, pacifism and universal connection is based.

The Liver and Gall Bladder Paired System

The Liver is prone to becoming damaged by the energy of the emotion of anger. This anger can either be outwardly expressed at others, or inwardly, so that it takes the form of frustration and self-hatred. Both inwardly directed and outwardly manifested forms of anger are equally damaging to the Liver, although outwardly expressed anger also has the potential effect of hurting others, especially when it leads to physical violence. The energy of the Liver also governs our tendency to compare our self to others and then to express negativity towards those we deem to be in higher positions than ourselves. These feelings of jealousy and a need to be perceived as higher than those around us are all energetic outbursts of the emotional energy of the Liver.

The emotional energy of the Liver is held in balance by the 'decision-making' organ: the Gall Bladder. If the Gall Bladder is functioning as it should then it will keep the self-destructive emotional outbursts of the Liver in check, enabling us to react calmly and sensibly to events and experiences we may have. It will enable us to see where the real roots of our feelings of anger lie, thus checking our behaviour before it hurts us and those around us, as well as the organ of the Liver. Figure 3.8 shows the emotional cognitive relationship of the Liver and Gall Bladder.

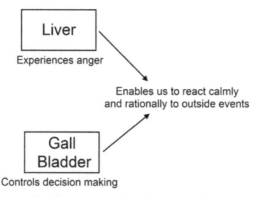

FIGURE 3.8: THE LIVER AND GALL BLADDER RELATIONSHIP

If we are to develop healthily as people and live successfully alongside others then we must balance the energies of these two organs. This will prevent us from looking outwards and comparing our self to others. This is the first step towards accessing the spiritual entity of the Hun which is anchored in us by the Liver organ.

THE CREATION OF PATHOGENIC ENERGY

The level of our emotional stability depends upon the state of equilibrium between the paired organs and how they continue to relate to each other. This balance is subject to numerous external and internal influences that may throw out this state of harmony; these can range from diet, environmental factors, emotional abuse and stress to predetermined conditions beginning at birth, to name just a few. As these different factors influence the paired organs, excess emotional energy starts to be discharged by the spirits of the organs themselves, resulting in negative emotional effects. This emotional energy then travels through the meridian system, giving it a direct interface with the entirety of our mind and body; it is at this stage that the energy of our emotions begins to affect our psychological well-being and physical health.

This energy travelling through the meridians will likely lead to stagnation and blockages in the various meridian pathways, which will contribute to the further development of disease. In more energetically based traditions of Chinese medicine these blockages were studied and mapped out, giving the Chinese medical practitioner an understanding of where to focus their attention in order to help clear the energetic blockage and thus help the patient back to health. From these theories they began to understand how different energetic pathways were connected to different organs and how certain meridian points were directly connected to different elements of the mind and body.

The organs give off a second form of by-product when emotional upset causes them to move away from a state of harmony. These by-products take the form of semi-physical energies which move inside the body to attack different tissues and areas of the body. It is easiest to think of these by-products as being like steam given off by an old machine when it is over-taxed. In letting off this 'steam' the organ is trying to protect itself from harm, but the very nature of the pathogen itself is damaging to the body. In ancient times these by-products were known as 'evil winds' and these winds (along with malignant spirits) were thought to be responsible for all internally based diseases. In contemporary Chinese medicine these winds were drawn into line with environmental pathogenic theory and adjusted to become the internal version of Damp, Heat, Cold, etc. By looking at how these by-products move inside the body and what form they take it is possible to see where Chinese medicine theory came from and to understand some of the reasons why certain organs are linked with other tissues, orifices and sense organs in Daoist medical teachings.

The By-Products of the Heart System

The Heart gives off excess Heat when it moves out of balance. Waves of warm, expansive Qi move out from the centre of the Heart when you experience an emotion such as joy or excitement or undertake an automatic action linked to the Heart, such as smiling or laughing. When you make the laughter sound 'ha, ha, ha' it is the Heart's way of letting off excess energetic Heat when you are experiencing joy. It is for this reason that many medical Qi Gong schools will have you chant the sound 'ha' repeatedly whilst performing a certain movement in order to help strengthen the Heart. They are matching the natural defensive sound that this organ causes you to make when it wants to vent Heat safely. Does this mean you should never smile or laugh? Of course not. It is natural and extremely healthy for the Heart to create this warmth and then expel it; this allows the expelled wave of expansion to move out from the Heart, positively affecting every aspect of your body. The pulsing wave of Heart Heat moves along the length of the meridians like waves on water, bringing positivity to the whole energy body.

Problems develop when there is either not enough Heat, as this leads to sadness and sinking Heart Qi; or too much Heat that is not being vented, so it becomes trapped. This trapped Heat can come from negative Heart-based emotions such as anxieties, nervousness or overly manic emotional patterning. The trapped Heat is known as Heart Heat in Chinese medical theory. This Heat begins to create warmth in the area of the chest, which the Pericardium will try to deal with. The Pericardium is a sack which surrounds the Heart, acting as a sort of energetic 'emotional buffer'. It takes this Heat and moves it away from the Heart itself and out through the length of the Pericardium meridian, which ends in the centre of the palms at a powerful meridian point known as Laogong (PC 8). This will cause the palms to begin to grow warm and sweat as the Heat leaves your hands. Most of us have experienced this at times when we were feeling anxious in some way.

When we smile and outwardly express joy this helps our Heart's Qi to gently rise and expand, bringing us good health. If we do not express joy, as in some cultures where it is actually frowned upon to smile, then the Heart's Qi will sink, leading to numerous internal problems.

If the excess energy being produced by the Heart becomes too strong due to being pent up for long periods of time, it will begin to turn into the pathogen known as Heart Fire. Heart Fire is the contemporary name for the energetic pathogen, the evil wind, produced by the Heart when it is in trouble. This pathogenic energy travels outwards and upwards from the organ of the heart, affecting other areas of the body as it goes. Figure 3.9 shows the movement of the energetic by-product of the Heart.

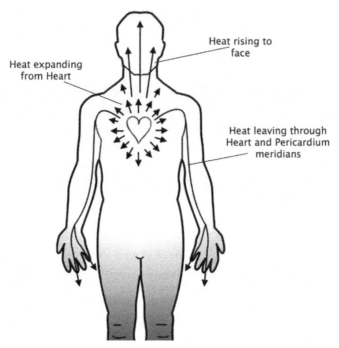

Heat rising to face

Heat expanding from Heart

Heat leaving through Heart and Pericardium meridians

FIGURE 3.9: HEART FIRE IN THE BODY

As shown in Figure 3.9, Heart Fire moves outwards to create excess warmth and imbalance in the area of the chest, neck and face. This can result in feelings of over-heating and redness coming to the skin in these areas. This redness often moves upwards into the face, leading to a person looking flushed all the time. The Fire affects the spirit of the Heart, the Shen, which becomes overly agitated, leading to a person developing anxious behaviour patterns and having an inability to be mentally or physically still. The eyes can begin to redden as the Heat enters them and they can begin to look slightly wild and staring in extreme cases; this would be known as a sign of the Shen being disturbed.

The pathogenic Qi from the Heart will move into the Heart meridian which originates externally in the centre of the armpit. Blockages here will result in swelling that can be quite painful to touch and usually feels warm. Redness and pimples can appear on the face and along the length of the Heart and Pericardium meridian, along with rashes and other skin eruptions around the area of the neck and face. This is the body trying to expel the pathogen through the meridian pathways and skin. Because of the internal pathway of the Heart meridian it is common for this pathogenic energy to begin creating mouth ulcers on the body of the tongue itself, although they sometimes spread into the rest of the mouth.

The By-Products of the Spleen System

The Spleen produces a pathogenic form of Qi known as Damp in contemporary Chinese medicine schools. This pathogen is a heavy, sinking form of Qi which moves down from the Spleen into the lower abdomen, where it gathers, leading to large amounts of stagnation. The stagnating effect of the Damp Qi in this region often causes fluid in the body to turn turbid, leading to an increase in body weight, generally around the midriff, although it can also spread around the rest of the body as well. Confusion often comes from the fact that a person can have Damp in their body but not have an excess of body weight; in fact they can be quite emaciated. In this case the Damp is still present, but rather than affecting the fluid mechanism of the body it is weakening the Qi mechanism of the digestive system that enables us to draw nourishment from our food. It is still common in these individuals to have a slightly swollen lower abdomen which is worse after eating, even though they may not generally carry a lot of weight on the rest of their body.

Damp pathogenic energy moves out from the area of the Spleen and sinks down and collects in the abdominal region of the body. A small amount also travels upwards, where it can cause a person's face to become slightly puffy, and some sticks to the diaphragm and lungs, affecting the breathing. Figure 3.10 shows this process.

This Damp can cause many problems, including making a person feel despondent, sluggish and heavy as their Qi begins to sink and coagulate. It can affect the bowels, which can become loose, and this often gets worse over time, leading to difficulties eating many types of food.

Damp is a massive problem in modern times as the majority of sugary, processed foods are very Damp forming. They directly attack the energy of the Spleen, so that it is highly likely to produce the by-product of Damp inside the body. This, combined with a lack of exercise, is largely responsible for the massive epidemic of obesity in the Western world.

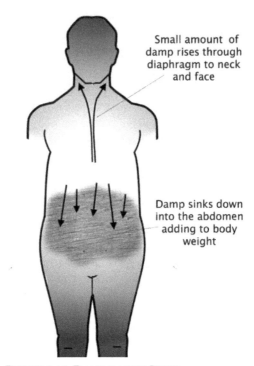

Small amount of
damp rises through
diaphragm to neck
and face

Damp sinks down
into the abdomen
adding to body
weight

FIGURE 3.10: DAMP IN THE BODY

The Spleen has a direct connection to the strength of the body's muscles, and so they can become flaccid and weak, resulting in a person feeling tired and lacking in strength. In the extreme this weakness spreads down the length of the Spleen meridian, leading to weakness and collapse along the inside of the legs and the arches of the feet as they react to the sinking Qi.

The By-Products of the Lung System

The Lungs like to be slightly moist, as this enables them to function properly and guide the distribution of fluids throughout the body (a function of the Lungs according to Chinese medical theory). However, an excess of this fluid results in the pathogen of mucus forming, which is detrimental of the health of the Lungs and our ability to breathe properly. Conversely, if the Lungs are not properly nourished with this fluid then they become overly dry and this also leads to problems.

If the Lungs are negatively affected by environmental factors or unprocessed feelings of loss and grief then the by-product of mucus starts to form. This pathogenic by-product is unique, as it actually manifests in a physical form which we can see when we sneeze or cough. It forms in the lungs themselves, the throat, the mouth, the nose and in our sinuses. It is these areas that become blocked and most negatively affected by mucus. Figure 3.11 shows this process.

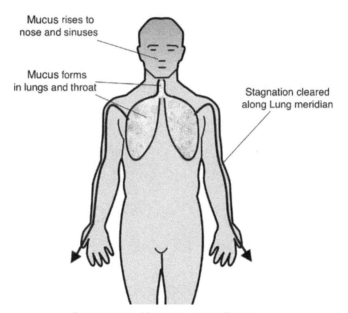

Mucus rises to nose and sinuses

Mucus forms in lungs and throat

Stagnation cleared along Lung meridian

FIGURE 3.11: MUCUS IN THE BODY

The Lungs open into the skin, which means that deficiency can lead to pale skin or even skin dryness if there is not enough fluid being formed. As the Lungs try to clear this issue they will try to expel the pathogen down the length of the Lung and the Large Intestine meridians. It is common for soft nodules to appear along the length of these meridians, which are easily felt if you palpate along their length. Tenderness and pain are also commonly present in the origins of the Lung meridian on the top of the chest around the Zhongfu (LU 1) points.

The biggest effect of trapped grief and sadness not being processed by the Lungs is tightness in the centre of the chest. The constricting nature of excess Lung energy overrides the expansive warmth of the Heart pulse, and the centre of the chest begins to tighten up and close. This causes the shoulders to hunch and the chest to collapse inwards, leading to pain and tension in the upper body as well as an inability to express joy properly.

The By-Products of the Kidney System

There are three main causes of Cold in the body. The first is a lack of internal warmth, meaning that the Cold is produced by weakness. The second source of Cold is from the outside world, as in the case of cold winter weather invading the body. The third source of Cold in the body is as a pathogenic by-product produced from the Kidneys when they are energetically and emotionally out of balance.

The pathogen of internal Cold is a gaseous form of Qi which collects in certain areas of the body causing contraction and tightness. It is a very draining pathogenic by-product which can lead to a person feeling very tired, as well as tense and immobile, both mentally and physically. Figure 3.12 shows the movement of the pathogen of Cold in the body.

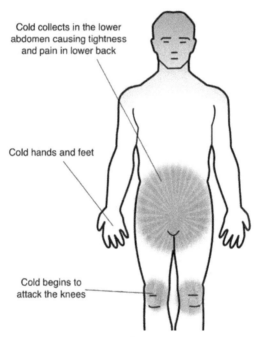

Cold collects in the lower
abdomen causing tightness
and pain in lower back

Cold hands and feet

Cold begins to
attack the knees

FIGURE 3.12: COLD IN THE BODY

The Cold pathogen causes the lower back to tighten, leading to lower back pain. If this is combined with low Kidney energy then the lumbar region will be particularly painful as the internal branch of the Kidney meridian in the lower spine becomes drained. This area of the body becomes cold to the touch, as does the lower abdomen just above the groin, which is where the pathogen of Cold travels next. This pathogen can also collect in the lower legs and knees, where the tightness can lead to leg pain, as well as in the extremities of the hands and feet which can feel cold to the touch. This should not be confused with the coldness in the body and limbs that can be experienced due to lack of warmth; this is an area of much confusion for anybody beginning their study of Chinese medicine, and one of the trickiest areas to diagnose accurately when you are new to the practice.

The tightness of the Cold in the body leads to a general contraction of the posture which may almost look as if a person is trying to huddle up with themselves for warmth when they are walking around. This may sound like an odd analogy but take a look at people walking around town on a cold day and you will understand what I mean.

All of this Cold in the body is directed by the emotion of fear and insecurity. It is these areas of the body that are most affected by the these emotions, and these feelings that will leave the psyche when Dao Yin training begins to free up the body's joints.

Along the length of the back runs the Bladder meridian, the organ paired with the Kidneys. This organ controls your emotional security and sense of self-worth. If this is attacked then the organ of the Bladder and your spine can become weakened and painful as the pathogen of Cold moves to this area of the body.

The By-Products of the Liver System

The Liver is subject to the emotion of anger and produces the by-product of Liver Gas as a result of this. In contemporary Chinese medical theory the concept of Liver Gas has been replaced by the concept of Liver Yang rising, but for Dao Yin theory we retain the ancient understanding. Liver Wind is a slightly different concept that you will often see discussed in Chinese medical texts but the theories are somewhat different. I personally find the Liver Gas theory to be very accurate when dealing with my patients.

The Liver gives off this Gas and it collects under the base of the diaphragm and in the intercostal spaces between the ribs on the sides of the torso. It causes the diaphragm to tighten, leading to shallow breathing which often sounds forced and as if it is coming from the throat rather than the chest. The torso can become restricted as the intercostal muscles tighten, leading to an even further detrimental effect upon the person's breathing.

The tightness of this Gas passes into the ligaments and tendons of the body that are governed by the Liver, causing the whole body to tighten and become very inflexible. This inflexibility begins to transfer to the mind, making it difficult for a person to see beyond his or her own belief systems and points of view. The Gas travels along the length of the paired meridian, the Gall Bladder meridian, so that the lateral twisting movements become difficult and the person's buttocks become tight, leading to tension in the hips and lower body.

If this Gas travels upwards then it can lead to migraine-type headaches and eye pain as it reaches the head. Figure 3.13 shows this process taking place.

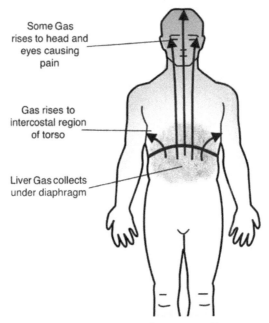

Some Gas rises to head and eyes causing pain

Gas rises to intercostal region of torso

Liver Gas collects under diaphragm

FIGURE 3.13: LIVER GAS IN THE BODY

Stress is one of the biggest negative influences upon the health of the Liver and Gall Bladder. Because stress is a non-obvious threat it does not necessarily lead to external outbursts of anger. There is no threat that can be perceived in the form of an actual person, so the pressure in the Liver just builds up over time. This leads to numerous health problems, including the symptoms described above, as well as a contraction in the Gall Bladder meridian. This meridian travels up into the shoulders and neck, so as it tightens it causes the shoulders and neck themselves to tighten. The first place that stress shows itself is usually in a person's neck and shoulders, as any massage therapist will tell you.

EXPERIENTIAL ENERGIES

So far in this chapter we have looked at the way in which the emotional and cognitive functions of the paired organs keep each other in balance. We have also looked at the pathogenic by-products that are produced in the body due to our emotional experiences. Now, in order to understand how this may manifest in our body we need to understand exactly where each of these pathogenic energies travels and sticks in the body.

A key aspect of the meridian system is that it stores information. Our energy body is like a gigantic library of each and every thing we have ever done. Every experience we have ever had is energetically imprinted into our system in the same way that our minds record these details through memory. Our consciousness and energy body are always looking to 'grow'. It is an innate tendency of human beings to want to evolve, not through inconsequential nonsense which we often believe betters us, like wealth and power, but through spiritual growth and adaptation. The energy body takes all of the information from our interactions and experiences and uses this to change us. In this way everything we do takes the form of a kind of energetic lesson, whether it is perceived as being positive or negative. This then adjusts the way we think, act and develop so that we literally become our own thoughts, beliefs and experiences. This is something of a double-edged sword, though, as some experiences steer us towards spiritual growth whilst others may hinder us and lead to an imbalance in our nature or well-being. The great argument is whether or not anything is good or bad. Classical Daoism would state that no such division exists, but for the sake of this book let us work to the assumption that the things that I refer to as negative are the things that are creating weaker physical and psychological health. In the case of many negative experiences it may be that we convert them to positive by learning from them, which enables us to grow, but sometimes, in the case of severe trauma or loss, this may be difficult.

Every interaction we have takes place on either a cognitive, communicative or physical level. This means that we experience this interaction using either one or more of our five senses, or simply with the mind, as in the case of our thought processes. At the same time there is also an energetic imprint of this event; this imprint carries information which is then stored somewhere in the energy body, changing us in some way. Some of this information is very precise, pertaining to exact memories of events, whilst other information takes the form of the pathogenic by-products discussed above.

Due to the nature of the meridian system and the location of these pathways through different areas of the body, it is possible to locate where different emotional and experiential pieces of information collect. For example, due to the connection between the emotions of anger and frustration and the Liver, we know that energy produced by these emotions generally travels in the Liver and Gall Bladder meridians. This means that it often sticks in the lateral region of the body, around the ribs and under the diaphragm, as well as around the buttocks and inside the hips. This information then leads to tightness and discomfort in these regions of the body, as well as potential physical ailments in the same locations.

This is relevant to Dao Yin training as the exercises are designed to take this information and purge it from the body. The extension of the mind out of the body combined with the movements and the special breathing method begins to lead this pathogenic Qi outwards. The aim is to get it to travel along the length of the meridian out towards the extremities, where it can be expelled. The result is that the energy body becomes clearer, the mind becomes quieter and the physical body will free up in the relevant areas. Long-term injuries resulting from pathogens in these areas of the body can improve and the joints can free up as the restrictive pathogens are expelled.

EMOTIONAL PATHOGENIC LOCATIONS

Figure 3.14 shows the front of the human body and the different areas where emotional energetic stagnation takes place. Figure 3.15 shows the rear of the human body.

As energetic information collects in these areas of the body, it can lead to the development of stagnation, which prevents healthy Qi flow. This results in tightness and the key Qi Men in this area becoming blocked. The effects of this are then cumulative; if old feelings of anger have begun to collect in the area of your ribs and create tightness, then Qi flow is now restricted through this region of the body. Gradually this blockage increases over time, which means that the anger is gradually affecting you more and more. The information stored here begins to change the way that your acquired mind works and so you will have a strong tendency towards feelings of anger in the future. Your past experiences are energetically changing the way you are, and so you are more likely to revert to this emotional standpoint in the future. Often when looking at the effects of energetic stagnation caused in this way we are referring to chronic unexplained pain which makes up a large percentage of people's daily discomfort. These are the long-term aches and pains for which there is no obvious medical explanation.

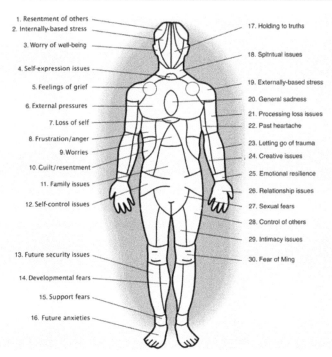

1. Resentment of others
2. Internally-based stress
3. Worry of well-being
4. Self-expression issues
5. Feelings of grief
6. External pressures
7. Loss of self
8. Frustration/anger
9. Worries
10. Guilt/resentment
11. Family issues
12. Self-control issues
13. Future security issues
14. Developmental fears
15. Support fears
16. Future anxieties

17. Holding to truths
18. Spitritual issues
19. Externally-based stress
20. General sadness
21. Processing loss issues
22. Past heartache
23. Letting go of trauma
24. Creative issues
25. Emotional resilience
26. Relationship issues
27. Sexual fears
28. Control of others
29. Intimacy issues
30. Fear of Ming

FIGURE 3.14: STAGNATION ON THE FRONT OF BODY

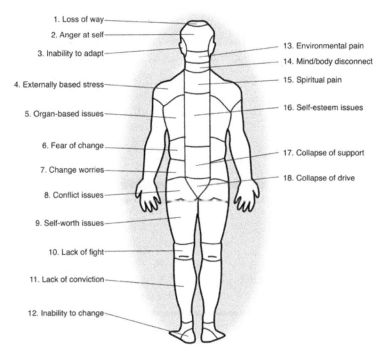

1. Loss of way
2. Anger at self
3. Inability to adapt
4. Externally based stress
5. Organ-based issues
6. Fear of change
7. Change worries
8. Conflict issues
9. Self-worth issues
10. Lack of fight
11. Lack of conviction
12. Inability to change

13. Environmental pain
14. Mind/body disconnect
15. Spiritual pain
16. Self-esteem issues
17. Collapse of support
18. Collapse of drive

FIGURE 3.15: STAGNATION ON THE REAR OF BODY

Now follows a discussion of each area of the body with regard to the emotional stagnation stored in that area.

Stagnation on the Front of the Body

The numbers next to each emotional imbalance correspond to the numbers on Figure 3.14.

1. *Resentment of others:* To feel resentment of others and their perceived position in comparison to yourself, and to feel frustrated or angry at how this reflects on your own sense of self, often leads to feelings of pain and stagnation in the temporal region of the head, moving upwards towards the top of the head. This can lead to migraine-type headaches as well. This stagnation travels up to the head via the Gall Bladder meridian, which is paired with the Liver meridian. This energetic pathway often carries the emotional by-products of the Liver.

2. *Internally based stress:* Stressful feelings due to pressures you put upon yourself to achieve or to live up to others' expectations are Liver-related energies which travel to the eyes, the sense organ closely related to the Liver. This results in eye pain, redness of the eyes and even redness and burst blood vessels in the eyes.

3. *Worry of well-being:* The Stomach meridian passes along the jawline. This meridian often carries emotional by-products from its paired organ, the Spleen. The energy of worry sits here; particularly worries over one's own level of health and well-being. If you are constantly worrying about your health and how it affects you, then the muscles of the jaw often become tense.

4. *Self-expression issues:* The Tiantu (Ren 22) meridian point sits at the base of the throat. This point becomes blocked with emotional stagnation when a person cannot express himself or herself fully, either verbally because they cannot find the words, or because they have been oppressed. This oppression of self-expression can be due to an uneven romantic partnership, an over-domineering parent or through extreme religious dictation. Stagnation often starts to develop here at quite a young age, weakening a person's voice and leading to physical problems in this area.

5. *Feelings of grief:* Emotional stagnation due to the loss of something or somebody you hold dear can begin to lead to tightness and

pain in the area of the 'shoulder's nest'. This is the origin of the Lung meridian, which is the key meridian linked to the emotions of sadness and grief. This tightness can cause pain, shortness of breath and a closing of the chest due to a tightening of the muscles in this area.

6. *External pressures:* Those experiencing a great deal of pressure to perform well will often develop energetic stagnation in the chest area. Note that this is different from the breasts in the case of women. This would be the musculature region beneath the breasts in the pectoral region of the body. Feelings of always having to be the best, be the strongest and lead others by example, cause stagnation in this region.

7. *Loss of self:* The solar plexus region of the body manifests the Earth elemental energy of creation. As we develop into human beings this energy moves out from our core. When it reaches the level of the solar plexus it manifests our own sense of self, and from here the Heart's energy is born, which gives us creativity and emotional feelings based upon this sense of self. If a person begins to lose who they are as an individual due to oppression from a loved one, parent, etc., then it is this area that will begin to stagnate. Note that there is a difference between a positive loss of 'self' through an experience of emptiness and a loss of sense of self through being manipulated into being somebody you are not. This stagnation is very common amongst people forced to compromise that which they hold dear due to a profession or vocation their parents and peers have forced them in to.

8. *Frustration/anger:* The upper area of the ribs under the arm store all of the pathogenic by-products of the Liver, which travel here through both the Liver and Gall Bladder meridians. When emotional by-products reach this area they lead to tightness and lack of flexibility. This causes 'bruise' type pain in the area of the ribs, which is also a positive indicator of the Liver's Qi flowing mechanism starting to stagnate.

9. *Worries:* The key place where we manifest the energetic stagnation of worries is in the upper abdominal region. This area then begins to tighten and feel uncomfortable. It can lead to swelling in the upper abdomen, which then spreads into the lower abdomen, leading to pain, abdominal distension and loose bowels.

10. *Guilt/resentment:* Feelings of resentment towards others will collect here as well as in the temporal regions of the head. Feelings of guilt about either wrongs you have committed against others or thoughts you harbour about others will also affect this area. These are more Liver-related energies which travel primarily through the Gall Bladder meridian.

11. *Family issues:* Most lower abdominal pain, stagnation, discomfort and physical problems related to this area of the body are a result of very deep emotional stagnation caused by the family. These issues are tricky to shift as they relate very closely to how a person developed from a young age when the parents and siblings were such an important developmental influence. This area is the physical centre of the body. It is this area that governs the 'life-giving' Earth elemental energy from which our physical body is born.

12. *Self-control issues:* Feelings of losing one's self-control or having a constant sense of having to 'maintain control' develop energetic stagnation in the hips. It is through this region of the body that the Gall Bladder controls the muscles of our hips, waist and the level of flexibility in our hips. When any negative feelings associated with the emotional energies of the Liver start to build up they must either be processed, expressed or repressed. It is repression of these emotions due to a need to maintain control that causes stagnation in this region.

13. *Future security issues:* The Stomach meridian governs this region of the legs. This is the meridian paired with the Spleen, which controls the emotional energy of worry. Worries about how best to progress into the future can develop stagnation, pain and nodules along the front of the shin.

14. *Developmental fears:* The pathway of the Spleen meridian along the inside of the lower leg is particularly prone to weakening if we have had any worries or fears around how we are developing. These can also be fears around our own sense of independence or how we were brought up as children. If we were 'over smothered' and not allowed to develop sufficiently on our own, then this area of the body can become weak and painful. This can lead to collapsed knees and fallen arches of the feet, as well as pain inside the inner leg radiating towards the knees.

15. *Support fears:* Any fears over our ability to support ourselves, either emotionally, energetically or practically with regard to finances and so on, can lead to stagnation, pain and weakness in the ankles. The energy of the Kidneys and Bladder is primarily responsible for the strength of the ankle microcosmically, which manifests the 'supporting' quality of the Kidneys.

16. *Future anxieties:* Fears around how the future will unfold and how we will cope with it can lead to stagnation, pain and weakness in the feet and toes.

17. *Holding to truths:* The front of our face pertains to the question, are we staying 'true' to ourselves? If we are constantly compromising our morals in order to survive, then it can lead to pain, stagnation and blemishes appearing on the face, particularly around the area of the mouth.

18. *Spiritual issues:* The head represents the kingdom of Heaven according to esoteric Daoist schools. The neck is the supportive structure that holds up the Heavens. It is for this reason that many of the meridian points that fall into the category of 'Window of Heaven' points sit upon the neck. Pain and stiffness in the neck shows disconnection from a sense of spirituality or a refusal to accept something we know 'deep down' to be spiritually true or poignant in our life.

19. *Externally based stress:* The shoulders manifest tension if we are stressed due to external events taking place in our life. This is probably the most easily recognisable stagnation for the majority of people. Tension in the shoulders shows itself as soon as we try to move them in any way. The Gall Bladder meridian has a key point here named Jianjing (GB 21), which means 'Shoulder Well'. It is thought that stress causes Qi to drop away from this point like water falling down a well, which leads to stagnation and tightness in the area of the shoulders.

20. *General sadness:* Any extreme feelings of sadness, either acute or chronic, will collect in the centre of the chest at a point known as Shanzhong (Ren 17). This point will gather up this sadness, which tightens the chest and collapses a person's posture inwards. It is very common for there to be a lot of tears when energy stuck in this area of the body begins to move.

21. *Processing loss issues:* The Lung meridian runs along the length of the outside of the arm, and so it is through this region of the body that any emotional disturbance generated in the early stages of dealing with loss or grief manifests. These energies stagnate here, leading to unexplained pain and weakness.

22. *Past heartache:* The inside of the upper arm is a very sensitive area both physically and energetically. Any emotional trauma that has strongly affected the Heart can stagnate in this area, leading to pain and increased sensitivity. If the Heart is regularly discharging through this region, then unexplained extra weight could start to form here as well. Most of these traumas seem to revolve around romantic relationships and most strongly affect women, in my own experience.

23. *Letting go of trauma:* In the final stages of letting go of loss, grief and emotional trauma it is common to have discomfort, tightness and even nodules in the lower arm. These usually clear by themselves but sometimes they get stuck and stay for a long time. This is all part of the Lung and Large Intestine's energetic function of transferring emotional traumas out of the body via their meridians.

24. *Creative issues:* The Heart likes to be creative; it is the organ of manifesting artistic expression. This is a natural and important aspect of human life. If this expression does not take place, then the lower aspect of the Heart meridian can become blocked, leading to pain and stagnation in this region of the body.

25. *Emotional resilience:* Many important 'source' meridian points sit in the region of the wrist. If we have a tendency towards a 'low emotional threshold', meaning that we are easily hurt and very emotionally sensitive, then there is usually some kind of pain, weakness or swelling in the wrists.

26. *Relationship issues:* The hands and fingers 'reach out to others' in Daoism. The fingers manifest our relationship to key people in our lives, including family and loved ones. Painful or crooked fingers are a representation of issues around key relationships, either past or present, in our lives. This is a very simplified way of looking at the hands, though; there is a whole study of palmistry and hand diagnosis in Chinese medicine which is beyond the scope of this book.

27. *Sexual fears:* Fears around sexuality and sexual expression often manifest in the groin and inside of the hips. This may be fear due to a negative sexual experience in the past, or fear because of guilt issues around expressing your sexuality. This is very common in homosexual people who are not fully able to express their sexuality if they feel threatened by others' views. Stagnation here leads to tightness and immobility in the hips.

28. *Control of others:* A feeling of superiority or a need to control others' thoughts and actions will stagnate in this region of the Gall Bladder meridian, leading to pain and tightness in this region. This immobilises the legs and prevents relaxation of muscles in this area of the body.

29. *Intimacy issues:* Our issues around intimacy, both physical and emotional, usually manifest as pain and tightness along the inside of the thighs. This emotional stagnation is often closely linked to sexual fears, so that stagnation here often radiates up into the area of the groin and hips as well.

30. *Fear of Ming:* Our Ming is our path through life, which we are helped along by the energy of the Kidneys. If we fear events or happenings which are coming up along this path then we will begin to develop emotional stagnation in the front and sides of the knees. The events we encounter along the path of our Ming are designed to help us grow as we overcome personal challenges. Understanding this helps to alleviate the fears, freeing up stagnation in this area.

Stagnation on the Rear of the Body

The numbers next to each emotional imbalance correspond to the numbers on Figure 3.15.

1. *Loss of way:* The top of the head is our connection to the divine. Through here the Chong Mai reaches up into the Heavens and gives us 'two-way' feedback between ourselves and the entity of Dao. Those who fully disconnect from this divinity will start to develop pain and stagnation on top of the head, as well as mood swings and many kinds of psychiatric disorders. This point is controlled by Baihui (DU 20) and the four protective points of the Sishencong (extra points with no number) which surround it.

2. *Anger at self:* Continued anger at your own thoughts, actions and speech will lead to stagnation developing in the Gall Bladder branches that run over the back of your head. This leads to migraine-type headaches and pressure at the back of the head, which begins to muffle a person's thoughts.

3. *Inability to adapt:* The pathway of our evolutionary meridian, the Triple Heater, runs around the back of the ears. This channel governs our ability to adapt to changing circumstances. If we are not able to, then it is common for aches and sudden pains to arise behind the ears.

4. *Externally based stress:* The shoulders manifest tension if we are stressed due to external events taking place in our life. This is probably the most easily recognisable stagnation for the majority of people. Tension in the shoulders shows itself as soon as we try to move them in any way. The Gall Bladder meridian has a key point here named Jianjing (GB 21) which means 'Shoulder Well'. It is thought that stress causes Qi to drop away from this point like water falling down a well, which leads to stagnation and tightness in the area of the shoulders.

5. *Organ-based issues:* Pain along here can be emotionally based but it is generally a more positive indicator of weakness in the various internal organs of the body. The 'Shu' points of the Bladder meridian, which will begin to ache if their associated organ is out of balance, govern this area. A quick look into any acupuncture book will show you which organ corresponds to each section of this area of the back.

6. *Fear of change:* The lower back around the area of the physical kidneys can begin to ache and tighten if emotional stagnation builds up here. This stagnation is normally due to the emotion of fear, which the Kidneys govern. This fear is usually around the concept of change, growth and development, which the Kidneys pertain to. It is also common for stagnation here to come with feelings of cold and low energy levels.

7. *Change worries:* If these fears of change develop into projected worries then stagnation will develop lower down in the midriff, leading to a gain of weight in this region. The Spleen has been weakened by your emotional state and so 'love-handles' may develop.

8. *Conflict issues:* Those who feel they must always 'fight' to survive will develop emotional stagnation in the buttocks, as the Gall Bladder meridian deposits the excess energy here. This marks an inability to relax, trust people and simply 'go with the flow'. Those who cannot understand that life is not always about fighting to get what you want will never manage to release stagnant pathogenic energy here and the buttocks will remain tight and clenched.

9. *Self-worth issues:* The region of the Bladder meridian which runs along the middle of the back of the upper legs governs our sense of self-worth. Those who constantly feel worthless in themselves will begin to develop pain and weakness in this area of the legs.

10. *Lack of fight:* Sometimes in life you must stand up for yourself in order not to allow others to affect you negatively. This is a part of life. If a person's ability to do this is weak then the Bladder meridian's energy running through the middle of the back of the knees will weaken, leading to weak knees, pain in the backs of the knees and tightness, which will radiate along the length of the legs.

11. *Lack of conviction:* The Bladder meridian branch running through the back of the calves governs our sense of conviction. Can we stand up for what we believe even when others ridicule us for it? Those who cannot, develop energetic stagnation in the backs of the calves, which may ache easily after exercise and will lack flexibility.

12. *Inability to change:* The heels are related to the water element's ability to flow and change. Water travels around obstacles and adapts to its environment; human beings need to do the same in order to develop healthily and the Kidneys and Bladder work together to help this happen. Those who cannot change often develop stagnation in the heels and pain underneath the feet which radiates along the sole.

13. *Environmental pain:* This is pain caused by environmental factors invading the body, such as extreme climatic conditions or pollution. Whilst the occipital region at the base of the skull has emotional correspondences to our spiritual health, it is difficult to make an accurate diagnosis based on the condition of this area, because it is also so affected by our environment. Any Cold or

Wind pathogens that enter the body have a strong stagnating affect upon this area of the neck.

14. *Mind/body disconnect:* As discussed earlier, the neck relates to our ability to connect to the divine energy of Heaven, manifested microcosmically in the head. The cervical section of our spine is the physical manifestation of this connection, and so any major disconnection between the mind and the body will lead to stagnation here. Tightness and pain quickly develop as the unity of consciousness and physicality is broken.

15. *Spiritual pain:* The upper thoracic spine pertains to our spiritual health. This is the region of the Shen, one of the key aspects of our consciousness. If our spiritual health is damaged in some way then the upper back will hurt. This can also be true if the Heart is damaged, as this is the residence of the Shen in the body.

16. *Self-esteem issues:* The spine is governed by the Du meridian and the Bladder meridians which run along the length of our back. They control our sense of self-esteem. Any issues around how we perceive ourselves will manifest here. If we constantly feel under attack and our self-esteem is damaged then the Bladder and Du meridians will want to protect us, resulting in a preference for lying and sleeping in the foetal position.

17. *Collapse of support:* The lower spine is closely connected to the health of our Kidneys, which are our energetic foundation. If extreme emotional difficulty has attacked us for too long then the supporting function of the Kidneys can become weakened and so the lower spine will hurt. This can be seen as the Kidneys energetically 'giving up'. The pathogenic energies that build up in this area from this process taking place must be cleared and new levels of inner resolve found in order to alleviate the problem.

18. *Collapse of drive:* In a similar way, the Kidneys also govern our drive, along with the Du meridian which governs the pole of Yang in our body. If these are damaged due to excessive emotional trauma then the sacral area of the spine can weaken as we lose our sense of drive. Pain will appear in the area right at the base of the spine and our motivation for engaging with life will greatly decrease.

EXPERIENCING THESE AREAS OF STAGNATION

An easy way to understand where exactly you are storing these emotional energies is to look at your physical weaknesses and structural imbalances. Where is your body tight? Perhaps you don't know. It is common for the body to try to hide these trapped feelings from you by normalising the way you feel so that you are unaware of your own level of discomfort. This is easy to see past though; spend half an hour stretching and moving your body in as many ways as you can, really push yourself. Now see where you are aching. Which parts of your body were tighter than the rest of your body? Did any bruised feelings arise whilst you were exercising? Is it clear that your shoulders are hunched or one is dropped? All of these can be used as diagnostic signs.

If you are generally quite internally aware then you may already be quite clued in as to where your problems are. You may well be aware of a tendency towards tightness in the body. Those unexplained bruise-like sensations that are not rooted in an obvious injury are quite possibly the result of emotional information stuck somewhere in your body. As stated above, most chronic, unexplained pain that people experience is a result of this kind of emotional pathogenic stagnation.

These theories are quite easy to understand if you are familiar with the layout of the meridian pathways and Chinese medical theory. When I work on patients using acupuncture, massage or Qi transmission it is often these areas that I work with. It never ceases to amaze me just how accurate these models are when working with people. Through massaging an area of the body or inserting needles into the relevant region area of the meridian system I am able to clear these pathogens. Almost as soon as it starts to clear, patients will start to release these emotions through crying, laughing or some other obvious emotional response. Others will open up and tell you everything about their lives and past traumas related to these areas of the body. All of these occurrences are signs of the stagnant pathogenic energy leaving the body. This is the same process that takes place through Dao Yin exercises, although, because it is an internal form of exercise and the patient is engaging with their own healthcare, I believe it to be stronger than any form of therapy you receive from an outside person.

CLEARING THESE PATHOGENS

The next step after understanding the nature and location of energetic blockages is understanding how to clear them. Of course there are numerous methods, but in this book we are focusing on Dao Yin exercises.

The next chapter discusses the principles inherent in any classical Dao Yin training, following which the four Dragon Dao Yin exercises are explored in detail. These exercises twist and pull open all the different regions of the body shown in Figure 3.14 and lead the stuck energies out of the body. The result of this is that you should find your body becoming more mobile, looser and generally more comfortable. These exercises greatly increase flexibility and joint mobility very quickly, but this is not just because of the way the body is moving. It is because pathogens are being purged from the energy body, which in turn frees up the Qi Men. This allows more energy to flow freely through the Qi Men area of the body, which softens the muscles. The muscles can now relax and elongate, which results in greater mobility.

A key factor in understanding Dao Yin exercises is understanding that the body does not want these pathogens stored in it. It naturally tries to expel them anyway and the effectiveness of this will depend largely upon the health of each individual. By practising Dao Yin exercises we are helping the body to expel the stuck energies that it wants to be rid of. You could think of it as giving the energy body permission to do what it wants to do anyway. This enabling of the body to be and function naturally is a hallmark of the Daoist tradition, which never wishes to force the mind or body into anything that goes against its normal function.

CHAPTER 4

DAO YIN PRINCIPLES

As discussed at the beginning of the book, Dao Yin exercises have certain qualities that make them quite distinct from the more commonly practised Qi Gong. Understanding these qualities and putting them into practice is what brings a Dao Yin exercise to life; without these principles a Dao Yin movement will be little more than a physical stretch.

The key principles of Dao Yin, which are discussed in this chapter, are the principles of extending the Yi, opening the Qi Men, lengthening along the Jing Jin and utilising Dao Yin breathing. Each of these principles should be applied universally across all Dao Yin exercises and certainly the Dragon Dao Yin sequences outlined in this book.

EXTENDING THE YI

The Yi is an aspect of human consciousness. It is one of the five spirits which are assigned to the five key Yin organs according to Daoist theory. The Yi is often translated as our 'awareness' or our level of 'mental focus' and it is the aspect of human consciousness said to reside in the physical organ of the Spleen.

The strength of the Yi and hence our level of mental focus is dictated by the health of the Spleen, which is the key organ involved in our digestive process in Chinese medical theory. If we have an unhealthy diet or our digestion is compromised in some way then our Yi will be negatively affected; in particular too many refined sugary foods are especially harmful to the Spleen and the Yi. An unhealthy Yi will result in a person not being able to concentrate properly, their mind will wander easily and it will be impossible to focus upon a task. Long-term imbalance in the Yi will lead to an overactive mind that cannot 'think straight', small issues can start to become over-burdensome and imagined issues are projected into the future, leading to inappropriate worrying. Everything is a problem and worries are not restricted to the individual; in time they will worry about everybody else, especially those closest to them, resulting in 'overbearing' and 'smothering' behaviour.

In all Daoist arts the strength of the Yi is very important as it is the aspect of mind that acts as a catalyst for the majority of internal processes to take place. We need to be able to rest our mind on various areas of our internal energy body and focus without becoming distracted, so that the 'Yi will lead the Qi' (a common phrase in Qi Gong communities). If we have excessive amounts of imagined worries that distract us from our work then we will never progress very far into the process of internal development. It is for this reason that relative stillness of the mind is important, along with a good diet. Any serious practitioner of the internal arts should regulate their diet to ensure the health of their Spleen and digestive system, as well as the general health of their physical body. If a practitioner ignores their diet and indulges in too much processed or sugary foods then the Yi will be unable to focus on the tasks required. A poor diet, which is based solely upon what a person enjoys eating, is not conducive to effective practice.

UNDERSTANDING THE YI

The Yi is very important in Qi Gong practice and can be understood by carrying out this simple exercise: Take one hand and extend your index finger as if pointing. Now look at the very tip of your finger and rest your awareness there. Just keep your mind there on the tip of your index finger for a few minutes and focus upon any sensations that may crop up on the tip of your finger.

Now, the exact point where your mind is resting and focusing is the point where your Yi is. I often explain it to students as being like a sort of set of 'cross-hairs' that are directed by the mind. Wherever your mind rests for a short space of time, this is the location of the Yi. If you focus long enough without letting your mind wander you will find that your Qi begins to move to this point, which is the reason for the Qi Gong adage 'The Yi leads the Qi'. After a short time you may even begin to feel the movement of Qi down to your fingertip. The sensation can vary from a slight temperature change and tingle through to a strong pulse or even a visual reaction of perceived light, depending upon your level of internal development.

The size and focus of the Yi can vary greatly, depending upon what goal you are aiming to achieve. It can either be focused to a very small point as in the above exercise, or it can be spread out, as in the case of gently observing reactions that are taking place across your entire body. It can also be gentle or it can be incredibly strong. The different strengths of focus will either gently cause Qi to flow to this area (in the case of gentle focus) or cause Qi to be led forcefully to the area and gather (as in the case of a strong level of focus). It is important that we understand the difference between the two strengths, as mistakes here are the reason for many Qi Gong deviations and sicknesses.

To understand the difference between the two strengths let us return to our previous exercise of focusing upon the index finger. First place your mind on the tip of your index finger and gently rest it there. You should feel as if you are 'gently observing' the end of your finger, as if you are only half interested in what is taking place there. The difficulty is that you need to keep this casual mindset whilst at the same time not letting your mind wander from this point.

If you keep your mind on the tip of your index finger in this manner for a few minutes you should start to be able to feel what the quality of the Qi movement is as it is led gently to the tip of your index finger. This experience will be slightly different for everybody, as each individual person's brain will interpret the experience slightly differently, and also experiences will vary according to natural levels of sensitivity and degrees of internal development. Whatever the experience is for you, make a mental note of it.

Now change the level of focus. Stare at the tip of your index finger and make your focus super strong. You should have the feeling of nothing else in the universe holding any importance at this exact moment, just the tip of your index finger. Hold your mind there and do not let it wander. Take mental note of any changes in sensation that take place after a few minutes of mentally staring at your fingertip in this manner.

This level of focus will strongly lead Qi to the area, where it will begin to gather, so it is common for your fingertip to feel as if it is beginning to swell, or for pressure to build up in this area; it is not always a comfortable sensation.

If you cannot feel the difference between these two levels of focus then I suggest you spend some time working on this practice as it is quite important to be able to distinguish between the two. As a general rule, when you have your mind resting somewhere inside the body, as in a lot of Qi Gong practices and many forms of meditation, it is wise to use a gentle focus. The focus needs to be soft so that the line is blurred between actually leading Qi somewhere and just watching while it does whatever it likes. This will enable the internal process to unfold for you but it will avoid the risk of leading to energetic problems which can be serious and very hard to repair. If you use the second level of focus, the very strong level, then Qi can move too forcefully, leading to damage to the meridians and high levels of internal stagnation. Many Qi Gong problems are caused by people being too intense with their level of Yi, thinking it will make them progress more quickly, or by those who cannot distinguish between the two levels. People who live in a constant state of stress due to their lifestyle or their nature will often revert directly to a very strong level of focus when they encounter Qi Gong, whilst thinking they are being gentle. As a teacher it is very important to be able to recognise these people and to work cautiously with them in order to prevent them from making dangerous mistakes in their training.

If we have our mind outside of the body, as in Dao Yin training, then it is fine to use a strong focus. It is beneficial as it helps the Qi to understand that it must leave the limits of your physical body and move out into the environment. This is what helps the energetic purging process to take place. There is no danger of any stagnation developing inside the body as the Qi is not being led anywhere inside of you, it is being led outwards where it can escape from the body. In Dao Yin training our mind is always outside of the body so that Qi can be encouraged to move in this way.

EXTENSION INTO THE DISTANCE

As discussed at the start of the book: if we wish to move Qi for a very small distance, then we need to extend our mind a long way. If we place our awareness just a few inches beyond the end of our fingers then it is highly unlikely that Qi will extend out of our body, no matter how strong our level of focus is. If, however, we focus a mile or so into the distance then our Qi is likely to begin to move out of us, probably still only a few inches, but that is enough to get the stagnant Qi out of our meridian system. It is for this reason that the most ideal place to practice Dao Yin exercises is outdoors with a far horizon so that you are able to extend your Yi a long way into the distance. The further away the horizon, the better.

It is easiest to achieve if you find an object in the distance, perhaps a tree or something similar. Stare at this object and place the 'cross-hairs' of the Yi onto this tree with a high level of strength and do not let your awareness waiver. Keep your Yi focused as you perform the exercises in the book, especially on the movements that involve a clear pushing movement.

Obviously, although this is the ideal, not everybody has the advantage of having a large space like this to practise and not everybody has access to open outdoor areas where they have relative privacy and a suitable climate. Growing up in Britain I got to know how frustrating it can be to wish to train outdoors and to have to put up with both wind and rain at the same time. No matter, it is also possible to practise indoors. You just need the largest space you can find, even if it only gives you a few metres of extension beyond the end of your fingers when you are performing the exercises. Neither the Yi nor the Qi is limited by physical structures, so if you have a strong enough mind you can extend beyond the limits of the walls of your house or training space into the distance and still get the same effects, albeit with a little more difficulty than if you were outdoors. The only thing to be aware of is not to extend out of your body into another person, as you can shift stagnant Qi information from yourself into another person very easily. Definitely do not practise in a room where there are small children or any pregnant women present, as they can be incredibly sensitive to any negative Qi. This goes for small animals as well. Whilst practising as a teenager and clearing a particularly stubborn blockage of toxic Liver Qi I managed to kill my mother's pet chinchilla. As I extended across the room I did not take its cage into account; there was a scrabbling sound, a squeak and then it flipped over and died. My mother was not impressed.

After you have finished practising, air the room by opening all the windows. Leave the windows open for a while and the stagnant Qi will be cleared by the fresh environmental energy entering the room.

This practice will seem particularly strange to those coming to Dao Yin from a background of meditation or Qi Gong, where a gentle inwards focus is combined with closed eyes to gain a completely different result. With practice, however, you will be able to distinguish between the two and you will notice the distinct feeling of Qi leaving the body along your line of extension, particularly when you exhale.

REPLACING THE PURGED QI

The biggest fear many students have when they encounter these practices is that they will be purging vital Qi from the body, which will leave them deficient in energy. There is no need to worry. Your Qi is leaving your body through these practices primarily when you exhale. You are 'breathing out' pathogenic Qi. When you inhale you will draw fresh environmental Qi into the body; this combined with the Qi coming up from the planet will ensure that you are replacing the purged Qi with healthy Qi. The shamanic nature of Dao Yin exercises means that this connection with the wider environment supports and nourishes the body during purging practice.

OPENING THE QI MEN

The Qi Men or 'Energy Gates', which were discussed earlier, are those energetic areas that sit in the joints of the body. These key areas of the body need clearing out through our Dao Yin training. This can only happen if we are able to open up the body and create space in the Qi Men while practising the different exercises.

The opening of the Qi Men relies on the effects of the Jing Jin lines being gently stretched open. The relationship between the physical and the energetic is absolute; this means that it is impossible to do something to the physical body without the energy body being affected as well, and vice versa. We can use this in our practice, as we can manipulate certain parts of our physical body in order to ensure that the energy body is doing what it is supposed to be doing during each exercise.

As discussed earlier, the Jing Jin acts as a kind of 'riverbed' for the meridians, which flow through the connective tissue of the body. If we correctly stretch out the Jing Jin then they encourage a certain direction of flow in the meridian pathways so that Qi can be directed in the body. As these lines of connective tissue open out they also exert a directional motive force upon the Qi Men such that any stagnant pathogenic Qi that is stuck in the Qi Men will be led outwards and can be expelled.

LENGTHENING ALONG THE JING JIN

The principle of opening the Qi Men cannot be separated from the practice of lengthening the Jing Jin. In order to fully lengthen and connect along the Jing Jin lines it is important that we understand a couple of details. First, the stretch that we are applying in these exercises must be even throughout. If you wish to stretch effectively all the way along a Jing Jin line of connective tissue then the power and length of the stretch must be even, all the way from one end of the Jing Jin line to the other. If the stretch is uneven then the muscles involved in the Jing Jin line begin to isolate from each other and Qi will no longer be effectively led to the extremities. Essentially this uneven engagement of muscles involved in the Jing Jin line is what is happening during exercises that involve contraction, such as excessive weightlifting and bodybuilding, which lead to stagnation of Qi rather than a smooth flow along the length of the meridian. Most Western forms of exercise would fall into this category, whereas Eastern forms of training such as the internal martial arts, Dao Yin exercises or yoga work towards correctly engaging and utilising the Jing Jin.

The second idea to understand is that we want stretching the Jing Jin to be gentle and relaxed, it must not be forced in any way. We are trying to encourage elasticity along the connective tissue, and overstretching is counterproductive when trying to achieve this, as well as being risky with regard to injuring the body. If you think of a rubber band and how it behaves when it is stretched you will understand the Jing Jin. If I gently stretch out an elastic band so that it has some power stored in it then it will spring back to its original shape when it is released. If, however, I stretch it right out to its maximum and hold it there for some time, it actually starts to lose some of its elasticity as the fibres of the elastic band become damaged. This is similar to what happens when the body is overstretched. If I continue with this practice for some time then the elasticity is gradually weakened more and more and the Jing Jin lines become torn and less efficient at guiding the lines of Qi which flow through them.

PUTTING THESE PRINCIPLES INTO PRACTICE

When practising these principles it is important to understand the nature of the body. Essentially your bones are quite solid and the rest of your body (when sufficiently relaxed) is quite soft. The bones are all held in place by ligaments and the attached muscles, and we can use this to our advantage. If we store tension in our body then the muscles will contract, causing the bones to move closer together, which results in the Qi Men becoming closed. As Qi tries to move through the Qi Men it gets stuck and begins to stagnate. Like water left standing in a pool for some time, it begins to fester, and this will then lead to poor health in the body.

If we can relax the muscles of the body then the muscles will be able to lengthen, the Jing Jin will open up and the bones begin to move apart, creating space in the Qi Men. The trick to doing this effectively is that we must open each of the Qi Men at the same time. If we are trying to direct stagnant energy along a particular Jing Jin line but one or two Qi Men are more open than some of the others on that line, then the 'unevenness' of the openings will cause Qi to stagnate once more. Figure 4.1 shows this principle.

Understanding this principle can sometimes be quite difficult and I see many practitioners of the internal arts stumbling over this block. It applies to arts such as Taijiquan, Xingyiquan and Baguazhang as well. If we cannot open evenly then the Qi cannot flow and internal force will never be gained.

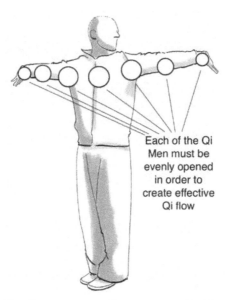

Each of the Qi Men must be evenly opened in order to create effective Qi flow

FIGURE 4.1: THE PRINCIPLE OF OPENING THE QI MEN SHOWN IN
ONE OF THE DRAGON DAO YIN POSTURES

Here is a simple practice to help understand this principle. When I teach my students I often find it useful to get them to practise it incorrectly first. Then trying it in the correct fashion allows them to feel the difference between the two.

Relax one arm and hold it out to your side as shown in Figure 4.2.

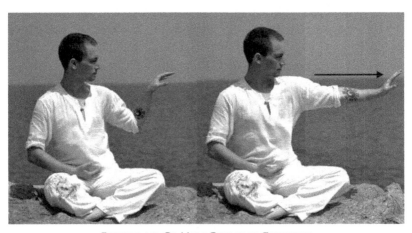

FIGURE 4.2: QI MEN OPENING EXERCISE

First, practise it incorrectly. Stretch out your arm into the distance as if you are trying to touch the furthest wall. Do not worry about how you do this; just extend your arm. Do this a few times and try to feel what is happening in your arms, and in particular each of the joints involved. These will be the joints of the shoulder, the elbow, the wrists and, if you are relaxed enough, the hands and fingers.

You are most likely extending with an emphasis on the hand. Generally when a person wishes to extend their arm their mind focuses upon the extremity, the hand, and the rest of the arm follows. This means that the muscles and connective tissue of the Jing Jin will open unevenly and the joints and Qi Men will usually remain closed. Whilst this may be fine for simple tasks such as reaching out to grasp an object, it is not the way we wish to move during Dao Yin practice.

Repeat the exercise but this time do not focus on the hand moving away from you. Instead, increasingly relax the muscles of your shoulder and arm and extend the arm more slowly. Focus on trying to create space in the joints of the shoulder, the elbow, the wrist and between the fingers, all at the same time, as you extend your arm. If one joint stops moving they all have to stop moving. If you can get the feel for opening each of the involved joints at the same time and to the same degree then you will begin to feel how we wish to open the body during Dao Yin practice. Mentally tune in to what it feels like to move your arm in this manner. It should feel quite different. It is quite common to feel rather bruised and tight the first few times you do this, as you are engaging different muscles from those you would normally use for such a simple movement. The shoulders may feel tighter than normal, as any habitual tension stored there will begin to show itself.

Try this exercise a few times and remember the feeling of moving your arm like this. This is the way we wish to carry out each stretching movement in Dao Yin practice. It can be quite tricky to do this with just your arm, so it can take even longer to manage it in the various twisting and opening postures of exercises such as the Dragon Dao Yin demonstrated in this book.

DAO YIN BREATHING METHODOLOGY

It is important for any internal practices that we understand how to use our breathing in the most effective manner. Our breath sits on the border between our energy body and our physical body; the air we breathe and the movement of our lungs have a direct effect upon the biological processes taking place in our body, but they also affect the movement of Qi through our body and control how smoothly this Qi flows. Since the aim of most internal practices at their core is to connect with and govern the movement of our Qi, it stands to reason that it is wise to spend some time making our breathing as effective as possible. I always recommend that any serious practitioner of Daoist arts should spend at least six months working on regulating the nature of their breathing, and then return to breathing exercises regularly over the years as their practice develops.

Remember that the key difference between standard Qi Gong exercises and Dao Yin training is that Qi Gong generally aims to regulate the flow of existing Qi in the body, whilst Dao Yin aims to move Qi along the length of a meridian and purge toxins from the key energetic centres that sit along the meridian's length. This means that different breathing methods are required for these different practices if we are to distinguish fully between the functions of Qi Gong and Dao Yin.

The vast majority of Qi Gong schools will begin by teaching deep diaphragmatic breathing whereby the breath is dropped low into the abdomen. This enables the diaphragm to expand fully downwards, which in turn helps the lungs to open to their maximum. It also directs the Qi downwards into the region of the Dan Tien, which is important for beginning any form of internal energetic movement. This form of breathing has a stretch on the lower abdominal muscles during inhalation and then uses a passive relaxation of these same muscles during exhalation. Breathing methods such as 'Sung breathing' or 'four directions breathing', which are common in many internal styles, would fall into this category. All of these breathing methods would be classified as passive or 'Yin' breathing methods. These breathing methods are fine and effective for Qi Gong training but for Dao Yin practice we require a slightly more Yang or 'assertive' way of breathing which engages the connective tissues of the body and our intention to a higher degree. This will help to shift Qi through the body to a greater degree and give us the ability to control the movement of pathogenic Qi out from the meridian system. In order to distinguish this form of breathing from other methods I will refer to it as 'Dao Yin breathing'. When practising any form of Dao Yin it is this form of breathing that should be utilised.

Dao Yin breathing is a form of abdominal breathing similar to Qi Gong breathing methods but it involves a small engagement of the lower abdominal muscles at the peak of the exhalation and extended use of the awareness or Yi in order to begin shifting Qi to a higher degree.

When learning Dao Yin breathing it is wise to work on some preparatory exercises first in order to prepare the body for this method. These preparatory exercises soften key muscle groups that are used for breathing and relax the diaphragm so that it can move more freely.

The process of Dao Yin breathing is as follows:

- preparing the body for breath work

- checking the fundamentals of breathing

- governing the inhalation

- controlling the exhalation in order to purge

- returning to Yin breathing.

I have the opportunity to meet a lot of different Qi Gong practitioners from around the world through the seminars that I teach, and it is very common for many people still to be struggling with their breath. Often the instruction that they have received is simply to breathe naturally, and no further instruction has been given. This would be a good instruction if everybody had healthy lungs, good breathing habits and a relaxed and well-conditioned diaphragm. Since this is often not the case there must be some work carried out on your own breathing habits in order to ensure that your 'natural' breathing is in fact correct and healthy.

Preparing the Body for Breath Work

Preparing the body for breath work involves ensuring that the correct muscles are suitably relaxed and springy so that they do not restrict our breathing in any way, as well as making sure that our inhalation and exhalation are smooth and even. This can take a little time to accomplish but through teaching I have seen the effectiveness of the small routine that I outline here. I generally get students to run through this a couple of times a week before they practise their Qi Gong or Dao Yin, and in a few months they find that their breathing has become a lot deeper and smoother.

The first thing we have to do is loosen the diaphragm. This large muscle extends across the middle of our torso below the ribs, effectively separating our abdominal cavity from our thoracic cavity. It is the key muscle used in respiration to allow the lungs to expand and contract efficiently. Providing that the diaphragm is healthy there will be a great deal of movement during breathing, as the diaphragm contracts and moves downwards into the abdomen during inhalation and then relaxes and moves up into the chest when we exhale, helping air to be pushed out of the lungs. Unfortunately most people have 'stuck' diaphragms that are restricted in their movements. This means that the lungs will not fully expand or contract, and when they do they often move in a somewhat jerky manner due to the areas of tension in the diaphragm itself.

The diaphragm sits in the centre of the torso as shown in Figure 4.3.

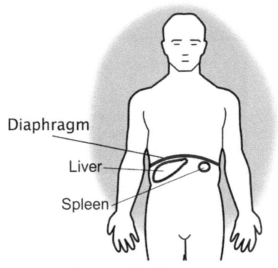

FIGURE 4.3: THE DIAPHRAGM

As you can see from Figure 4.3, the diaphragm is situated directly above the spleen and liver as well as other internal organs. This is important because of the pathogenic by-products that are released by these organs when they are not in balance. These pathogenic factors are actually forms of Qi which then have further detrimental consequences for the body's internal environment. The Spleen produces a form of Qi known as Damp in Chinese medical terminology and the Liver produces a Gas which was classically known as an 'evil wind' in ancient Chinese medicine, but in contemporary Chinese medicine it is often overlooked. These pathogens were discussed in detail in Chapter 3. As these pathogens move onto the diaphragm they cause it to stiffen through contraction. This contraction tightens the muscle and so our breathing becomes compromised. One of our first tasks is to clear the diaphragm of these pathogens and return it to a healthy and useful state. We can do this through a couple of simple exercises and a basic self-massage exercise.

Preparing the Diaphragm

Sit cross-legged on the floor, or on a chair if you are unable to sit on the floor comfortably. Now lean over to one side with one hand on the back of your neck, as shown in Figure 4.4.

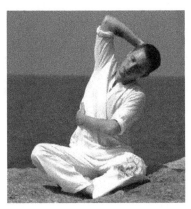

FIGURE 4.4: POSTURE FOR BREATHING INTO THE DIAPHRAGM

Take your opposite hand and place it on the side of your body where the ribs end, so that you can feel under your palm the lower part of your ribcage where the edge of the diaphragm would connect. You should aim to stretch the ribs and side of your body open as depicted. Take a few deep breaths into this area of your body, aiming to stretch the diaphragm open. You should feel the area of your side underneath your palm expanding strongly as you inhale into this region. When you inhale in this way you are stretching the edge of the diaphragm from the inside, using your lungs. Providing that you have no lung weakness or damage to your ribs or the muscles in this area, it is okay to breathe in with a little force at this stage in the exercise as you are simply aiming to expand the lungs enough to stretch the muscles in this area. Repeat this exercise on the other side of your body.

Now we wish to expand the front of the diaphragm, which sits along the line of the front of the ribcage as this is the key area that gets stuck through Liver Gas, Damp from the Spleen or trapped emotional information, which often sits in the area of the chest.

Lean back just a little so that the front of your body is stretched open. It should not be so much that it causes you discomfort or compresses the lumbar region of your spine. Place one of your hands on the front of your body under the edge of the front of your ribcage and spread your palm as shown in Figure 4.5.

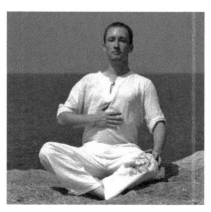

FIGURE 4.5: STRETCHING THE FRONT OF THE DIAPHRAGM

In the same way as in the previous exercise, breathe into your palm and aim to stretch open the area of your torso that sits under your palm. This will stretch out the front of the diaphragm. Aim to breathe with a little power into the area under your hand but do not be surprised if you miss the first couple of times. It is actually quite difficult to breathe directly into this area of the body, as the lungs like to expand either above or below where your hand lies. It can take a few goes to breathe accurately into your hand. Breathe like this a few times to help fully stretch out the diaphragm.

The next stage in our preparation is to help relax and return elasticity to the intercostal muscles which sit between our ribs on the sides of our torso. It is common for these muscles to become tight and restricted over the course of our daily lives and a simple self-massage practice can help with this. In many Qi Gong traditions it is said that you should not breathe with your ribs and that your intercostal muscles should not be utilised in any way; this is simply not the case. Your body is designed to breathe using the entire body and the ribs play a major part in the respiration process. In the internal arts we generally breathe down into the abdomen and so there is a large degree of expansion in the lower abdominal area. This ensures that the diaphragm extends fully downwards, creating space for the lungs as well as ensuring that the lower Dan Tien is fully stimulated as we breathe. This means that movement and use of the ribs and intercostal muscles becomes secondary, but it is still present. To aim to keep the ribs completely still when we breathe is essentially unnatural for the body and will lead to energetic and physical stagnation in the upper torso. Remember that in the Daoist arts we should never engage in anything that is unnatural for the body.

Running through the area of the ribs are the Gall Bladder meridian and the Liver meridian. These are the meridians of the Wood element, which are negatively affected by the emotion of anger along with frustration, annoyance and guilt. Any excess experience of these emotional states causes the Qi in these meridians to stagnate, which in turn tightens the muscles that sit along the length of these meridians. The intercostal muscles are some of these key muscles and experience has shown me that the upper intercostal muscles are mainly involved in feelings of repressed anger or frustration, and the lower intercostal muscles are generally tightened through feelings of guilt. Figure 4.6 shows this on the body.

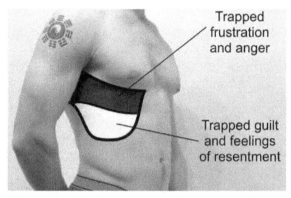

FIGURE 4.6: THE INTERCOSTAL AREA OF THE BODY

In order to massage the intercostal muscles and help free them of stagnation we need to make the hand shape shown in Figure 4.7. We extend the knuckle of the index finger and support this finger with the thumb. In Chinese martial arts this fist shape is often known as the 'phoenix eye fist'. It helps us to direct all of our force down to the single extended knuckle in the same way that a drawing pin ('thumb tack' in American) enables the power of a person's thumb to be focused to the tip of a small spike. This is going to be our massage tool.

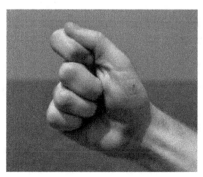

FIGURE 4.7: INTERCOSTAL MASSAGE HAND SHAPE

Take your knuckle to the opposite side of your body and massage deeply along the line of the ribs in the spaces between them where the intercostal muscles sit. If you have no injuries or weaknesses in this area then feel free to add the other hand for support so that you massage more deeply into the tissues of this area of your body. You should run the knuckle of the thumb along the spaces between the ribs as shown in Figure 4.8 and work into the tension. If you think of rubbing the silver layer from a scratch-card you will get the idea of how you should be using your knuckle.

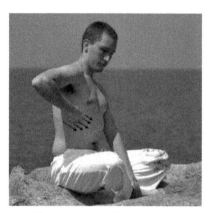

FIGURE 4.8: MASSAGE AND DIRECTION ALONG RIBS

Do not be surprised at the amount of physical discomfort this can produce at first. Pain is simply a by-product of stagnation according to Chinese medical theory, and so any stuck energy along the Liver or Gall Bladder meridians will cause this area of the body to become tender. This is all of your trapped guilt and pent-up frustration. Gradually as you repeat this massage you will find that the pain eases up and you will feel freer as the stagnation leaves the body. The intercostal muscles will also become more relaxed, which means that they can enable the lungs to expand more and so your breathing will improve.

Now place your hands on your knees and twist your body slowly in both directions several times. Have the intention of turning from your centre where the diaphragm sits. Twisting in this way helps to loosen the muscles of your core which connect into the respiration process. Figure 4.9 shows these twists.

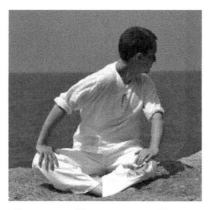

FIGURE 4.9: TWISTING THE TORSO

Now finish your breath work preparatory exercises by taking several long, deep breaths in and out through the nose, allowing your diaphragm to expand fully downwards into your abdominal cavity. Ideally take a few minutes just to relax and breathe. If you are familiar with the 'Sung breathing' process then this would be a good time to practise for just a few minutes. If you are not familiar with 'Sung breathing' then just continue to breathe deep into the abdomen.

Checking the Fundamentals of Breathing

Breath work has always been a major part of any internal system and so over the centuries spiritual practitioners around the world have carried out a great deal of study into the process of respiration. In the Daoist tradition it was seen that the more effective you could make your breathing, the more efficiently you could contact and work with your body's Qi. Once we have prepared our body by stretching the diaphragm and loosening any muscles on the torso that may be preventing us from fully expanding our lungs, it is wise to check through the absolute basics of abdominal breathing in order to ensure that we are practising correctly. When teaching breath work I have often seen the same errors popping up time and time again. Whilst they may appear to be small mistakes, adjusting them can greatly improve the quality of your breathing and thus your connection to the energy body. The key factors we must assess and, if necessary, correct are the length and smoothness of the breath, the use of the correct abdominal point and the use of the nose in breathing.

SMOOTHING THE BREATH

A common analogy for the meridian pathways of Qi in classical Daoist texts is that of water. The movement of energy along the channels in our body is likened to rivers and streams flowing through us. Many of the names of meridian points reflect this image of moving water, and key energetic centres where Qi collects and pools are often named after lakes, marshes and ponds. The metaphor of water works well for us if we want to understand exactly how our breathing affects our energy body. If the meridians are like waterways, then our breath is like the wind which blows across the surface of these waterways. A heavy, coarse breathing pattern will produce waves and choppiness in the water, whilst a gentle, smooth, even respiratory pattern will help the water to flow gently along the meridians. If we wish to expel power suddenly and harshly then a sudden, controlled use of sharp breath expulsion will produce a powerful surge which is much like waves crashing on the rocks. This kind of breathing is studied and used extensively in the internal martial arts where Qi is used to strike an opponent.

Even if we use the occasional powerful breathing method to make our Qi surge, we still want our regular, unconscious breathing to be smooth and even, so that our 'resting' Qi flow is smooth with no roughness to it. If we are able to make our breathing even and smooth then our Qi will flow smoothly, whilst a rough, uneven breathing pattern will lead to the gradual development of stagnation, the energetic basis for many forms of disease. Figure 4.10 shows the different effects that our breathing patterns will have upon the flow of Qi in our meridians.

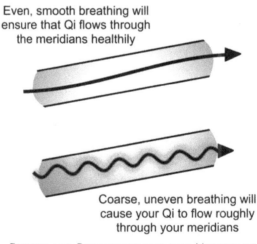

Even, smooth breathing will ensure that Qi flows through the meridians healthily

Coarse, uneven breathing will cause your Qi to flow roughly through your meridians

FIGURE 4.10: BREATHING AND THE MERIDIANS

Begin to look at smoothing out your breath by relaxing into a comfortable position; this can be sitting as in meditation, standing or even lying down. Relax your eyelids until your eyes close, and begin breathing gently in and out through your nose. Spend a few minutes just relaxing and breathing like this with no real focus to your practice. Just observe what is taking place in your body as you breathe and get used to your regular breathing habits. After a few minutes begin to observe the inhalation; this is the time when your ribs expand and your diaphragm moves downwards into your abdomen. When you inhale, your lungs expand and stretch inside the thoracic cavity, meaning that inhalation is the least passive part of breathing. If you have spent some time working on the intercostal muscles and stretching the diaphragm then you should have no problems breathing in nice and deeply, which helps to oxygenate the body fully and bring Qi from the environment into the meridian system. Most people find that the inhalation is much easier to regulate than the exhalation. The key thing you should be checking here is that the strength of your inhalation is even throughout. There should be no 'stuttering' in the lungs when they expand and there should not be a feeling of gasping for air. Gasping is quite rare but I have observed it in students who are going through emotionally difficult periods of their lives. If this is the case for you, then take some time just to observe these patterns and you will find that the attention you are giving your breathing will begin to cause it to change on its own. If you have problems with your inhalation then this needs to be your priority, as poor inhalation will lead to poor nourishment of the body with regard to oxygen and environmental Qi.

It is far more common for people's exhalation to need improving. I have observed that most people actually use a lot more force at the beginning of their exhalation; this force then gradually eases off towards the end of each exhalation, resulting in a hiatus before the next inhalation takes place. The over-emphasis on force at the beginning of the exhalation results in a slightly choppy nature to the flow of Qi through the meridians. There are two reasons for the excess of force at the start of each exhalation, which are (1) the intercostal muscles are tight, or (2) there are emotional tensions causing the chest to push the air out of the lungs. Both of these issues can be improved by taking control of the exhalation and working on consciously smoothing out the breath; this will in turn help to flex the intercostal muscles and relieve the mind of emotional stress.

Focus on the exhalation as you practise your breathing. Try to feel if there is any particular part of your body that feels tight at the peak of your inhalation. Is this tightness causing an excessive 'squeezing' of the lungs at the beginning of your exhalation? Is this squeezing causing air to rush out quickly? If it is, then it means your breathing will become quite feeble towards the end of each exhalation, as there is less air in the lungs and the muscles of the body are not as stretched out. Take control of the exhalation for roughly 10 to 20 minutes and ensure that you do not allow this excessive squeeze to take place. At first it can feel a little awkward but with time and consistent practice your body will understand what it is supposed to do and your exhalation will become smoother and more even. Do not be surprised if, with 20 minutes a day of this practice before you go to bed or in the morning, it still takes around six months or so before the breathing becomes very smooth all of the time. It is not always a fast process to regulate your breath.

Many people who practise Qi Gong have had the experience of feeling their Qi in the fingertips or hands. Beginners are often pleasantly amazed at the feelings of static and buzzing in their hands as they begin to connect with the exercises they are learning. What they are actually feeling, though, is the choppy nature of their Qi flow. The buzzing feeling could be likened to those rough waves in the flow of the meridians as the Qi is unevenly forced through the channels by unregulated breathing. If the breathing, particularly the exhalation, is smooth then these buzzing feelings of Qi should vanish, and instead the hands and fingers should pulse pleasantly in time with the breath. It can feel a little like the arteries pulsing with blood pumped by the heart, although much slower as the Qi is led by the breath rather than the heart.

USING CORRECT ABDOMINAL POINT

When we inhale whilst abdominally breathing our diaphragm should stretch downwards, enabling the lungs to fully expand. The front part of our abdomen also expands, in particular the lower abdominal muscles below the navel. The lower back will also move but this generally begins to take place on its own, providing you are breathing correctly into the lower abdomen as described here. There are different opinions on which point of the lower abdomen we expand and breathe into, which generally range between the navel itself, the meridian point known as Qihai (Ren 6) and the meridian point known as Guanyuan (Ren 4). These points are shown in Figure 4.11.

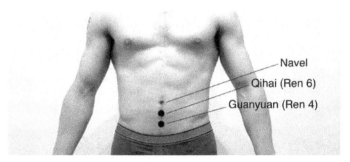

FIGURE 4.11: LOWER ABDOMINAL MERIDIAN POINTS

In my opinion it is most efficient for our practice to breathe into the Qihai (Ren 6) point. If you wish to feel why, then take your index finger and place it onto each of the three points shown in Figure 4.11. Now take a few deep breaths, aiming to fully expand the lower abdomen into each of the points in turn. Examine your body and feel what is taking place as you breathe into the points.

- *The navel:* Breathing into the navel means that the lower abdominal muscles are expanded unevenly with an emphasis on the upper abdominal muscles. The diaphragm tightens on the front of the ribs and the Qi does not sink fully down towards the lower Dan Tien region of the body. As a result the breathing should feel as if it sticks higher than in the other two points discussed here. Those with a high level of internal sensitivity will also find that the temperature of the lower Dan Tien gradually drops as you breathe into the navel, as it causes Qi to move away from it.

- *The Qihai (Ren 6) point:* Breathing into this point means that the emphasis on the expansion of the lower abdominal muscles is evenly spread. The space created in the abdomen should fully enable the diaphragm to expand downwards, which will in turn lead the breath and Qi down towards the lower Dan Tien. This should feel like the smoothest point to breathe into and create the most comfortable feeling on inhalation. The name of the Qihai point means the 'Sea of Qi' which refers to its close connection to the flow of Qi emanating from the lower Dan Tien itself.

- *The Guanyuan (Ren 4) point:* Breathing low into the abdomen into Guanyuan unevenly emphasises the lower abdominal muscles, meaning that tightness is created in the sides and rear of the diaphragm. This restricts the breath and prevents the breath and Qi being effectively being led into the lower Dan Tien.

Once you have settled on which is the most effective meridian point to breathe into, spend some time just gently breathing and training your diaphragm always to expand downwards towards this point. If every time you begin any Qi Gong or Dao Yin practice you just stand or sit and breathe into this point for a couple of minutes, it will not take your body long to learn that this is how it should breathe all of the time.

The Nose in Breathing

It is common for beginners in the internal arts to breathe through their mouths. This is incorrect for a couple of reasons. First, the nose has numerous tiny hairs which are designed to filter the air as you inhale, preventing damaging material from entering the lungs. They also help to warm the air as it enters your body, which does not happen so effectively when you inhale through your mouth. Exhaling through the mouth has the effect of 'diffusing' the internal pressure, rather than controlling it as the air leaves the nostrils. The diffusion of internal pressure means that the energetic field is not encouraged to expand fully as you exhale.

Most important though, and often missed, is the fact that the nostrils cause the Qi led into the body to spiral as you inhale it, whilst Qi brought into the body via the mouth does not do this. This happens because of there being two nostrils. Two points of entry for the Qi in the environment mean that the two sources of Qi twine around each other and spiral as shown in Figure 4.12.

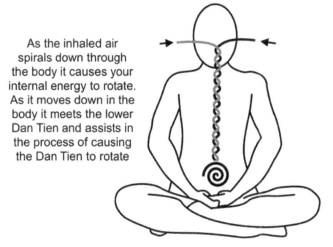

As the inhaled air spirals down through the body it causes your internal energy to rotate. As it moves down in the body it meets the lower Dan Tien and assists in the process of causing the Dan Tien to rotate

FIGURE 4.12: SPIRALLING THROUGH THE NOSE

This spiralling energy is led downwards into the body as you inhale, causing the Qi of the lungs to swirl. This helps to manifest the energy of Taiji in the body, which assists in moving Qi in an enlivening manner throughout the rest of the meridian system. When intermediate to advanced stages of internal practice have been reached it is possible to feel how this spiralling energy moves not only into the lungs but down into the lower Dan Tien on inhalation as well.

When you inhale in the Daoist arts you wish to ensure that your nostrils flare slightly to create more space and allow more breath into your nose. This can take a little practice but after a while it becomes automatic and does not take any conscious effort.

It is also useful before beginning breath work to seal off one nostril by pressing it shut. Take a few breaths in and out through the open nostril and then repeat the exercise on the other side. This just ensures that both are open and involved in the breathing process during your exercises.

THE DAO YIN BREATHING METHOD

The Dao Yin breathing method is a form of abdominal breathing which is very similar to the standard breathing method utilised in the majority of Qi Gong systems. It has one key difference: it is more Yang, as it has a less passive exhalation. There is a gentle engagement of the lower abdominal muscles as we exhale to help direct the exhalation from the region of the lower Dan Tien. This assists in driving the Qi in the meridians with a little more power, helping to lead it out to the extremities.

The first thing we need to understand about Dao Yin breathing is that, although it is still quite gentle in comparison to some other breathing methods used in the Daoist arts, it must not become our standard breathing method. By this I mean that we should only use this method of breathing at certain times when we are aiming for certain goals, such as during Dao Yin practice. Once we finish our practice then we should ensure that our breathing returns to regular, passive, deep diaphragmatic breathing as discussed earlier in this chapter. This ensures that the energetic circulatory effects of passive, Yin breathing are maintained throughout the course of our daily lives, helping us to remain calm, relaxed and healthy. The more Yang Dao Yin breathing exerts more drive onto the Qi moving in the meridian pathways, means that it can be useful in short bursts whilst we are practising. However, it should not be maintained for several days or more as it will lead to a slight over-excitement of the energy body, which can lead to hyperactivity and heightened emotional states.

Over the years that I have been training in the Daoist arts I have practised numerous different breathing methods. There are so many different ways to work with the breath and each is designed to achieve a certain aim. Some are highly effective and some others are very risky. I have seen people do themselves great harm with the more forceful breathing methods such as 'reverse breathing' or 'fire breathing'. The trick is never to underestimate the strength of your breathing. It directly governs the quality of your Qi flow and so will have an effect on every aspect of your mind and body that your Qi governs. Problems arise when practitioners do not spend time to gain control of their breathing, which means that they are not able to switch between the different modes at will. Their regular, unconscious breathing becomes changed from Yin diaphragmatic breathing to one of the more forceful methods, and so they begin to overexert their energy body, leading to internal damage. It is simple to avoid these issues; just make sure that you practise enough to gain control of when you are using certain breathing methods and return your unconscious breathing back to normal after each practice session. If a teacher does not ensure that you are doing this and does not give you time to return to your usual breathing method after each practice session, then they are being reckless and running the risk of causing you to hurt yourself.

Warnings aside, Dao Yin breathing is not as powerful as some of the other techniques mentioned above, so many of the risks are not applicable. It would take a long time of breathing in this way to develop any major problems.

Governing the Inhalation of Dao Yin Breathing

Inhalation for Dao Yin breathing is the same as for regular Yin abdominal breathing, with one exception. We inhale as far as is comfortable and natural and then we expand the lungs and abdomen just a little more. This extra inhalation creates a little pressure in the abdominal region of the body due to the extended stretch of the lungs, which helps to generate a little more pressure from the contraction of the abdominal muscles as we exhale. This extra little 'push' creates a stronger drive through the meridians as we exhale.

All of the principles for inhalation discussed above apply here, so we ensure that we have loosened the diaphragm and intercostal muscles as much as we can before we practise, we breathe smoothly with no 'jerkiness' and we ensure that we inhale through the nose down into the correct point on the lower abdomen. For regular, Yin abdominal breathing it would be enough just to inhale until we naturally feel we wish to stop. For Dao Yin breathing we need to inhale until we just begin to feel a little stretch in the lower abdominal region. This stretch should be subtle and not too much. Excess force will lead to stagnation of Qi in the abdomen, so inhale and keep going until you only just feel that the abdominal muscles begin to feel stretched. This means your inhalation will be only slightly deeper than when you are breathing with regular abdominal breathing.

Controlling the Exhalation in order to Purge

When exhaling using Dao Yin breathing, we need to ensure that, as discussed above, we even out the power of the exhalation throughout in order to ensure that we do not have all of our power at the start of the breath, in which case the end of each exhalation becomes quite feeble. This is very important; if you are not yet comfortable with this principle then return to working on this to ensure that it is fairly easy and takes place unconsciously in your breathing. If this principle is not in place then Dao Yin breathing will be too difficult for you and you will run out of breath before the end of each exhalation. This means that the Qi will not be successfully driven through the meridians, weakening the effects of the Dao Yin exercises.

In order to create the extra push of the Qi which is required for Dao Yin training we need to use the lower abdominal muscles like a second diaphragm. They need to be engaged slightly at the end of each exhalation to help drive the Qi out towards the extremities. When this breathing method is combined with the action of the lower Dan Tien and the extension of the Yi, it is fairly simple to make Dao Yin exercises work as they should and they quickly become a powerful form of purging.

For the exhalation it is important that we are able to control our lower abdominal muscles. Place your hand on the lower abdomen just below the navel and breathe in and out a few times. Do not worry about specific points as earlier; instead just try to feel the movement under your palm. Now, as you finish your exhalation add a little push from the muscles beneath your palm. This push should be very slight, as the lower abdominal muscles contract ever so slightly. It is important that we do not overdo this push. It should be very slight with only the 'suggestion' of a push, so that we give the idea to the Qi that it is supposed to move outwards from the centre of our body.

This push with the lower abdominal muscles needs to be smooth and still adhere to the principle of keeping the exhalation smooth and even throughout. This might sound impossible, as you are adding force with the abdomen, but remember that by the end of the exhalation your diaphragm will have finished relaxing back into its rest position. This means that the diaphragm is no longer assisting the lungs in the exhalation process, so we just substitute for it with the 'second diaphragm' – the abdominal muscles.

As you breathe in this manner you will find that the length of your exhalation increases, and after a while you will feel your Qi reach the end of your extremities. The power of the internal push is greatly increased when you get used to breathing in this manner.

At first you may find that you feel a little breathless after each exhalation as a result of fully expelling the air from your lungs. This may have happened because you have pushed too excessively. Relax a little and ease off on the power, as you have most likely expelled all of the air from your lungs, resulting in an almost 'gasping' quality to the start of your next inhalation. Remember that being gentle is the key. If you practise for a while with this breathing method isolated from any movements it will not be long before it feels natural and smooth.

Those who also practise Nei Gong, specifically Dan Tien work, should not be surprised if this breathing method causes the feeling of the lower Dan Tien turning over at the end of each exhalation. It can even cause your lower body to jerk a little as the Dan Tien affects your lower abdomen. This is because the push at the end of the exhalation exerts an increase in internal pressure in the lower abdomen and hence the lower Dan Tien as well. It is all part of the process for purging the energy body and is quite natural.

Returning to Yin Breathing

After any practice of Dao Yin breathing or indeed the Dao Yin exercises from this book, make sure you return your breathing to regular, Yin, abdominal breathing. Take a few minutes to either sit or stand quietly and practise your regular breathing. Ensure that there are no extra stretches on the inhalation or pushes on the exhalation, as these tools are no longer required.

After returning your breathing to normal, relax, shake out your body and walk around for a few minutes to let everything settle.

SUMMARY OF DAO YIN PRINCIPLES

The principles discussed here can take some time to get used to, especially if you have previously only studied an art such as Qi Gong, which is much more passive in nature. You should really practise all of these principles until they feel natural and easy enough to put into practice. Once you have managed this then you can start to combine them with some Dao Yin movements. This will result in the process shown in Figure 4.13.

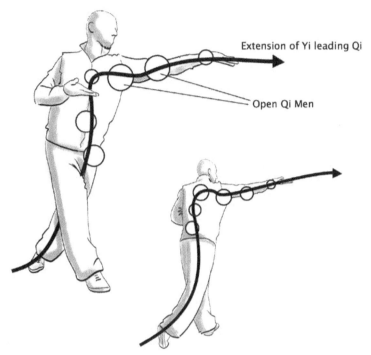

Extension of Yi leading Qi

Open Qi Men

FIGURE 4.13: DAO YIN PROCESS

This image shows how this process would be applied to a posture from the first Dragon Dao Yin exercise, which is covered in this book. This posture is shown from the front and the rear. You can see how during this particular movement, which emphasises a strong twisting movement across the whole of the body, a number of the key Qi Men energy centres are open. This provides a clear pathway through the energy body, through which Qi can move when the Dao Yin breathing method is applied. With the addition of a strong point of focus which extends the Yi into the distance, the energy in the meridian system should begin to move. This leads pathogens out of the body along the line shown in the image. If you compare this diagram to the chart showing where different emotional pathogens stagnate in the body (Figure 3.14), you can see how it helps to clear out several of these areas. These pathogens will then be led out of the body, producing a higher state of mental and physical health.

HARDWIRING IN THE INTERNAL ARTS

Though it is a modern term, 'hardwiring' is a phrase that has been absorbed into many internal arts schools. It refers to the process of gradually layering principles into an external practice such as a form or sequence. To try to practise the Dragon Dao exercises immediately with every one of the above principles would be practically impossible. You would end up very confused and your energy body would not know what to do. Each principle has to be gradually layered into the practice, ensuring that each has been fully absorbed before you progress. If you try to layer on a new principle before the previous one has been understood on an experiential level, then your foundation will be weak and neither principle will work effectively.

The process of hardwiring can be seen in any art such as Dao Yin, Qi Gong or Taijiquan. Beginners start with the body movements and then gradually their teacher adds a new principle. At first this is usually a breathing method. Once the breathing has been correctly performed then it is time to add another principle, such as the intention. This process then continues until a practitioner understands the full repertoire of principles inherent within whatever they are doing. An art such as the Dragon Dao Yin exercises must be learnt in this way in order for them to come alive. Each principle in this book must be added one layer at a time.

The problem with this is that most students of the internal arts will want to move too fast. I can fully relate to this problem, as when I was younger I was always wanting to move ahead. I had little patience for developing at the correct speed and gave my teachers constant headaches. Now I have learnt patience and see the sense in progressing at a correct speed for hardwiring. Because I did not learn at the correct speed in the first place, I have had to 'backtrack' in my practice a great deal and hardwire in each stage one at a time. I would have saved time if I had been less enthusiastic in the first place and ensured that I had each principle in place before I moved on. As a teacher you will often find that a student feels that they have incorporated a principle correctly long before they actually have. This is particularly common in those students who come to you with a great deal of prior experience in other arts. It is the job of the teacher to ensure that you do not teach at the speed a student wishes to learn, but at the speed they need to learn in order to understand what they are doing. If you are learning from a book such as this one then you must exercise restraint and patience and really ensure that each stage has been fully integrated into your core before you move on.

If you can successfully understand this process then you will move deep into your art. Though it may seem like a slow way to progress, it is actually the fastest route, as those who don't understand the hardwiring process properly will, at some point, hit a glass ceiling that they cannot move past.

CHAPTER 5

BEGINNING DAO YIN
THE FOUR WALKS

Now that we have looked at the development of Dao Yin, the nature of energetic stagnation and the qualitative properties of Dao Yin, it is time to start learning some actual exercises. In this chapter I will introduce the most fundamental of the Dragon Dao Yin exercises, the four walks. Each of these exercises is a form of Dao Yin which is practised whilst walking in a straight line, with the exception of the fourth, which 'zigzags' to some degree. These four walks have been isolated out of the sequences that they are a part of as I have found it easier for people to learn the exercises in this way. It is also a fact that almost all of the purging properties of these exercises exist in the walks. This means that if you are interested solely in increasing your mobility and learning how to purge the energy body, there is really no need to learn any exercises other than those in this chapter. The intermediate stage of learning all four entire sequences is only for those either looking to go deeper or looking for more of a personal challenge.

The four walks are named as follows:

- Piercing Palm

- Dragon Plays with Pearl

- Flying Dragon

- Drunkard Walking

Each of these four forms is described and examined below. It is wise to learn the movements first as empty shells. Treat them as nothing more than physical movements until you understand the co-ordination involved in each exercise. Then gradually begin to add in the various principles from Chapter 4 in order to bring the exercises to life.

DRAGON DAO YIN WALK 1: PIERCING PALM

Originally these exercises were a part of the Baguazhang system of martial arts. They were a form of body conditioning or 'Ji Ben Gong' which showed a martial artist how to access the correct muscles and lines of connective tissue so as to develop power effectively in one of the style's key techniques known as the 'Piercing Palm'. Gradually the exercises were extracted from the Baguazhang system due to their incredible health benefits and practised as medical exercises. Dao Yin principles were applied to them and they became effective forms for clearing out the energy body. When this happened the emphasis on effective power for combat was no longer required, so the exercises were adjusted a little. Despite this, the first walk retains its name of Piercing Palm as homage to what its original aim was.

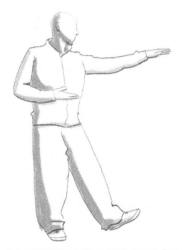

FIGURE 5.1: STARTING THE PIERCING PALM WALK

When starting the walk it is customary to begin with your left side forward and your left arm extended. If you are going to go on and learn the entire form from the next chapter then it is wise to get used to starting on this side of the body, since the sequence will put you in this position.

All of your weight is in your right leg at this time and your left leg is slightly extended. There should only be a slight bend in your right, supporting leg as this walk does not require much of a 'squat' into your legs. Your right hand rests on your centreline with your hand open, just beneath the level of your Heart or middle Dan Tien. The palm is facing upwards. Your neck should be extended and your head held high to ensure that the spine is not collapsed. Your left arm should be gently extended with the palm facing downwards. At this point you should be relaxed, with a gentle feeling of opening the joints being applied to the whole body.

Before beginning the first Dragon Dao Yin walk you should relax here for a few minutes and breathe gently. Let your mind become quiet and try to forget everything about the outside world; the only thing that matters at this particular moment is the exercise in hand.

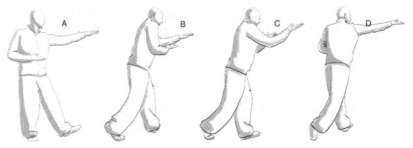

FIGURE 5.2: PIERCING PALM WALK (1)

Figure 5.2 shows the first stage in the Piercing Palm walk. The sequence shown in these four images would constitute one movement.

Your left foot should currently be without any weight on it, as you are in the starting posture shown in image A. Now shift your weight into this leg and twist outwards on the heel as shown in image B. All of your weight should now shift to the left leg and the ball of the right foot should be pressing lightly into the floor so that the Yongquan (KI 1) point is being stimulated. This helpfs to draw energy from the planet up into the body. Begin to slide your right hand underneath the left as you rotate your centre. Try to move the entire body in a smooth circle, as if your pelvis was a large wheel turning you around a single point.

Continue this turn until you reach the position shown in image C. At this point the right arm has continued to extend whilst the left hand is being withdrawn. The left hand also begins to turn over to face the sky at this point.

Continue turning until you have fully extended your right arm and withdrawn the left back to your centreline, underneath the level of your Heart or middle Dan Tien. This should put you in the position shown in image D. It is at this point that you fully extend out the joints, opening them to affect the Qi Men within them. You should also try to feel that even stretch along the whole body as the Jing Jin lines are lengthened.

This entire movement should be carried out on an exhalation with your Yi extended far into the distance. The speed of the movement can vary to some degree but it should be dictated by the speed of your exhalation.

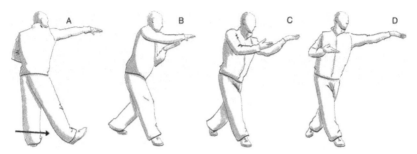

FIGURE 5.3: PIERCING PALM WALK (2)

Figure 5.3 shows this same movement being carried out on the opposite side of the body. The only confusion can come with the initial step being taken in image A.

In order to change to the other side of the body you must begin by stepping through with the rear leg, as indicated by the arrow at image A. At this point you also turn over your extended hand so that it is now facing the floor. Essentially you are moving back into the starting position shown in Figure 5.1, only this time you are on the opposite side of the body. As you make this small step and turn over your lead hand, you inhale and relax the stretch from the last posture.

Now repeat the instructions from Figure 5.2, only in reverse so that you are moving through the same exercise on the opposite side of the body. This should be fairly simple if you have managed to do it on the first side of the body. Again, this is all done on an exhalation, with your Yi extended into the distance. Finish the movement by opening the Qi Men and stretching out the Jing Jin once more.

If you can do this then you have completed two steps in the Piercing Palm Dragon Dao Yin walking exercise. Do not worry if they feel complicated and quite clumsy right now; it can take some time before they feel natural but with some practice you will get there. These two movements can then be repeated as many times as you like, depending upon how much space you have in front of you. In the parks in China it is very common to see people practising walking Qi Gong and Dao Yin through the length of the entire parks, which are usually fairly large.

The aim of this movement is to put a strong stretch throughout the length of the entire body whilst opening the key Qi Men around the areas of the chest, spine, shoulders and arms. The effect is much like wringing out a cloth. You should be able to feel exactly which Qi Men are opening during this exercise but, just in case, Figure 5.4 shows the key areas of the body you should aim to open when performing the Piercing Palm Dao Yin exercise.

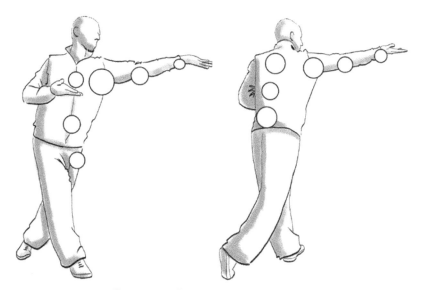

FIGURE 5.4: PIERCING PALM QI MEN

Once you sense that you are beginning to get a feel for the movement then gradually begin to add in the different layers of Dao Yin principles. This is what makes them such efficient exercises.

DRAGON DAO YIN WALK 2:
DRAGON PLAYS WITH PEARL

The second walking Dragon Dao Yin exercise is known as 'Dragon Plays with Pearl' and it is from the 'Swimming Dragon' sequence. The name should not be confused with the energetic principle of 'Dragon Plays with Pearl', which refers to the combined action of the Chong Mai and the lower Dan Tien rotating, rather than an actual set of exercises. This movement is simply named after that principle.

This movement, like the Piercing Palm exercise, is based around taking small steps forward whilst moving your spine and arms in a certain way. It can also be practised for as many steps as you have space in front of you. The starting position for this exercise is shown in Figure 5.5.

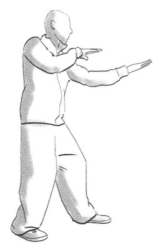

FIGURE 5.5: STARTING THE DRAGON PLAYS WITH PEARL WALK

Stand with your left foot slightly forward, as this is the position you would be placed in if you were performing the entire Swimming Dragon sequence. Your weight should be placed evenly between both feet, as with this exercise you are mainly concerned with rotating the body around your centreline and not so concerned with twisting the body's core as in the Piercing Palm exercise. Your right arm should be gently extended with your palm facing upwards. Your left arm should be lightly withdrawn with the palm facing downwards. When practising the Dragon Plays with Pearl exercise it is important to keep the palms facing each other whilst we perform the movements; this means that one will always be facing the sky and one facing the floor. Your hands should both be extended in front of you on your centreline.

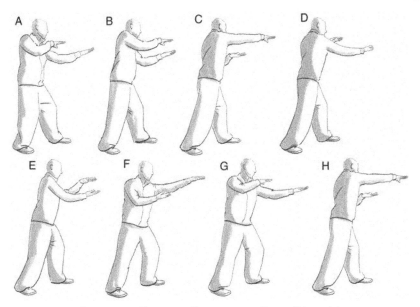

FIGURE 5.6: DRAGON PLAYS WITH PEARL WALK (1)

When performing the exercise we are going to move our arms three times in a 'rolling' fashion before stepping forward. Throughout we should try to keep the feeling that we are rotating a ball between our hands and rolling it up and down the length of our arms.

Turn the waist and extend your right arm outwards whilst retracting your lower left hand. This is shown in images A, B and C. It is at this point that you try to keep the image of rolling a ball between the arms. The smoother you can make this movement, the better. Once you have done this you will have completed the first of three arm movements.

Now switch your arms around so that the extended right arm drops down to become the lower arm and the left arm rotates upwards to become the upper arm, as shown in image D.

Repeat the process of turning your waist and switching your arms, so that the left arm now extends forward and the right arm retracts back in towards your body. This is shown in images E and F. This is the second arm movement of three.

Once more switch the arms over, so that the left arm is now on the bottom and the right arm is on the top. This is shown in image G. Finish by repeating the first movement of extending the right arm outwards and retracting the left arm. This is shown in image H. You have now completed the three arm movements which should be carried out before taking a step forward.

It is important that your breathing is correctly linked with your movements in order to maximise the purging effects of the exercise. You should begin by exhaling whilst extending your arm for the first time as shown in images A, B and C. You inhale through images D, E and F and then exhale again through images G and H. This means that you will be exhaling whilst you are extending the arm opposite to the leg you have in front. In this case, this means you exhale whenever the right arm goes forward, as you have your left leg in front.

It is important that your Yi is extended far into the distance when you extend your arms. The emphasis on cleansing is on the exhalations, so this is the most important time for you to extend your Yi.

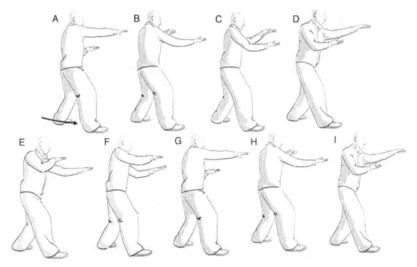

FIGURE 5.7: DRAGON PLAYS WITH PEARL WALK (2)

In order to walk forward in this exercise we simply take a small step forward, as shown in image A of Figure 5.7. This should leave you with your right foot forward and your right arm extended. Once again you should have your weight evenly distributed between your feet, as is the case for the whole of this exercise. You should inhale gently as you take this step.

Figure 5.7 shows the same exercise of Dragon Plays with Pearl being performed on the other side of the body, with your right foot forwards. This should be fairly easy to do, but remember that your exhalation takes place when you extend the arm opposite to the foot you have in front. On this side of the body it means that exhalation will be on extension of the left arm.

Once you have started to get used to this way of walking and moving, you should try to generate the movements from the correct part of the body. The Dragon Plays with Pearl is primarily aimed at opening the Qi Men at the base of your spine and rotating the point where your lumbar vertebrae connect into the pelvis. This means that you should aim to twist and turn your body from the waist whilst generating the arm movements and stretching of the Jing Jin from the base of your spine. This can take some practice but once you manage it you will have an effective exercise for clearing stagnation from the lower spine, the area of your Kidneys and the length of your back. Figure 5.8 shows the primary Qi Men which are opened up by the Dragon Plays with Pearl exercise.

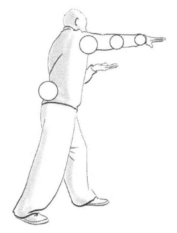

FIGURE 5.8: DRAGON PLAYS WITH PEARL QI MEN

Once you have a feel for the exercise, begin to gradually integrate the various Dao Yin principles discussed in Chapter 4 of this book. This will help the exercise to come alive and have a strong internal function.

DRAGON DAO YIN WALK 3: FLYING DRAGON
The third Dragon Dao Yin walking exercise is known as the 'Flying Dragon'. It is the most effective of the four exercises for opening the Qi Men around the area of the neck, chest, front of the abdomen and the shoulders. It is based around a very common upper body conditioning exercise which is featured in most styles of the martial art Baguazhang. It is also sometimes practised in some styles of Taijiquan and Qi Gong, where it is commonly known as the 'tea-cup exercise'.

This exercise is quite a jump in complexity from the first and second Dragon Dao Yin walking exercises, and so it is wise to learn the arm movements in isolation from the legs when you are starting out. Figure 5.9 shows the arm movements from the Flying Dragon exercise.

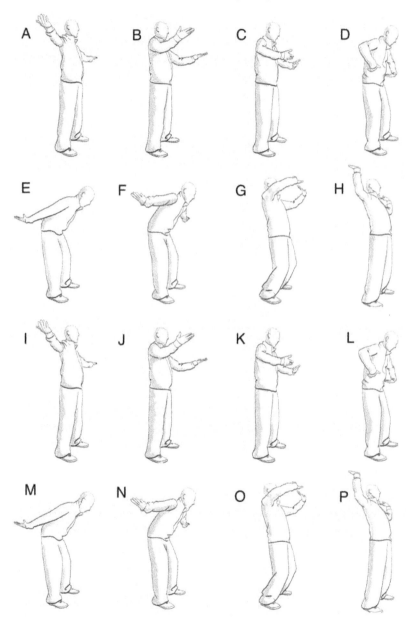

FIGURE 5.9: FLYING DRAGON ARMS

Stand naturally and begin in the position shown in image A. Your arms should be relaxed and gently extended. Begin the exercise by bringing your arms around and in towards your armpits as shown in images B, C and D. Your palms should be facing the sky as you do this. Now push your arms back behind you as shown in image E. The arms then come around and over your head as shown in images F, G and H. This should enable you to circle your arms around to the starting position shown in images A and I. This movement is then repeated, as shown in images J–P. These circles can then be linked together into one continuous exercise which works open the chest and shoulder areas of the body.

This exercise can seem tricky at first, but it is fairly easy so long as you remember to keep your palms facing the sky. At no point in these movements should your hands turn away from facing the sky. The exercise is sometimes known as the 'teacup exercise', as a classical way of learning this movement was to place a full cup into the students' hands and have them repeat the movements. If the cup was dropped or any fluid spilled then they had performed the movement incorrectly; feel free to give it a go but do not use your best tea set!

Throughout this exercise you should simply breathe naturally and relax the muscles of your upper body as much as possible. Do not be surprised if this movement quickly makes your shoulders ache a great deal. The movement causes you to make pretty much every different movement your shoulders are capable of making, so any tension stored between your joints and under the scapulae will show itself very quickly.

A common mistake with this exercise is that students circle their arms with the emphasis on the arms following the movement of the hands. This should not be the case; instead the movement of the chest should lead your arms and hands. You need to relax your upper body and create every movement from the centre of your chest whilst the arms and hands stay completely relaxed.

You should practise this movement until it is smooth and natural before beginning to take it to the next level and combining it with the stepping movements.

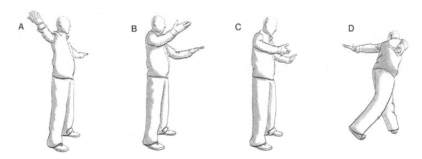

FIGURE 5.10: STARTING THE FLYING DRAGON WALK

In order to begin combining the Flying Dragon arm movements with the stepping, you should be in the position shown in image A of Figure 5.10. Your palms are facing upwards and you are standing with your feet at shoulders' width apart. Begin to bring your arms in towards your armpits as shown in images B and C as you fully inhale.

Now take a small step forward with your left foot; initially place your heel down and then rotate on the heel as you twist your body around to the left and look over your left shoulder. Shift all of your weight into the front foot as you do this. The Yongquan (KI 1) meridian point of your rear foot should be pressing down into the ground in order to help bring energy from the planet up into your body. Your arms extend out from underneath your armpits and stretch behind you as you lean slightly forwards. All of this is carried out on an exhalation and should leave you in the position shown in image D.

If you can complete this movement successfully then you are halfway there to learning the Flying Dragon walk. Most students find this the most intricate of the four walks with regard to body mechanics, so do not worry if you struggle with this one at first. The key is to remember that no matter how complex it may initially look, you are essentially just performing the previous arm movements whilst stepping forwards and twisting your body.

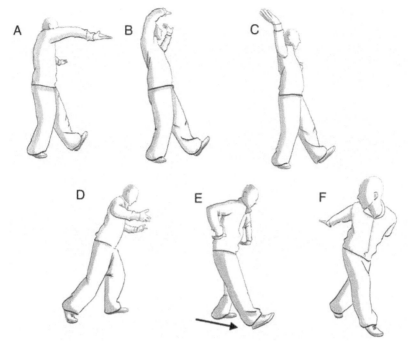

FIGURE 5.11: FLYING DRAGON WALK (1)

Starting from the previous position, we are going to begin by shifting our weight back into the rear leg by slightly leaning our body. As we do this we lift the toes of the front foot and look slightly up towards the sky. Our arms circle around from behind us with the palms still facing the sky, and we bring them around to above our head as shown in images A and B of Figure 5.11. Continue the circle of the arms around into position C. All of this is carried out whilst inhaling.

As the arms come around and our hands are in front of our armpits we shift our weight back into the front foot and begin to exhale. This is shown in image D.

Image E shows the point in the exercise where we take a step forward with our rear leg. As always, I have marked the step forward with an arrow to make the exercises easier to follow. We should adhere to the principle of keeping each step empty as we place our foot down. This means that our heel lightly touches the floor as we step forward and we ensure that it is in the correct position before we commit our weight forward into this leg. This is a stepping principle common to many forms of Qi Gong and arts such as Taijiquan. Energetically it means that the rocking to and fro of our weight stimulates the Yongquan (KI 1) point.

Finish the walk by shifting your weight into the front foot as you rotate around the heel and twist your body around to the right, as shown in image F. Look over your right shoulder as you fully extend your arms backwards and open up your chest. This completes the first step of the Flying Dragon walking exercise. Take some time and repeat this many times until you are able to complete one full step of the Flying Dragon walk. If you need to go back and isolate the arm movements, then feel free. It is wise to take your time and make sure each stage is fully understood before you try to move on.

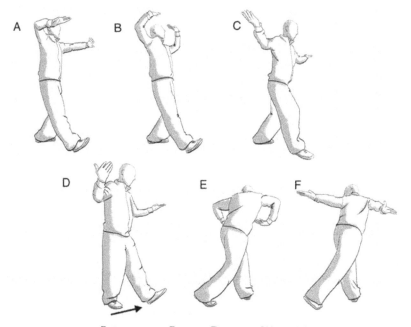

FIGURE 5.12: FLYING DRAGON WALK (2)

We now repeat these movements on the other side of the body in order to continue with the exercise. Figure 5.12 shows the sequence on the opposite side of the body. Pay close attention to the weight shifting back in image A, the step forward in image D and the completion of the exercise with the full twist in image F. Inhalation takes place during images A–C and exhalation is from images D–F.

Keep working on making the movements smooth and even, with no obvious hesitations or breaks in the circling of the arms. The speed of the movement should be dictated by the speed of your breathing, which can sometimes be slow and sometimes fast; feel free to explore the different feelings of the exercise when performed at different speeds.

If you have successfully followed the instructions for the Flying Dragon walk up to this point then you have completed two steps of the exercise, one on each side of the body. As with the previous walking exercises, these steps can be linked together for as far and as long as you like.

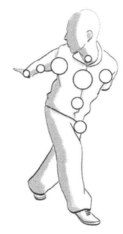

FIGURE 5.13: FLYING DRAGON QI MEN

Figure 5.13 shows the key Qi Men which are opened through performance of this exercise. The Flying Dragon is mostly for opening the Qi Men on the front of the body, neck and shoulders, although it does also work the entire spine. Experience has shown me that this exercise is very powerful for correcting postural issues in the upper half of the body. Bones often click and crack as beginners work on these movements!

As with the previous exercises, keep practising the Flying Dragon walk until you are comfortable with the movements. Once you feel that you are starting to get to grips with them, begin to integrate the various Dao Yin principles from Chapter 4.

DRAGON DAO YIN WALK 4: DRUNKARD WALKING

Although it may seem an unlikely image for classical martial arts to use, there are numerous styles based around the actions of being drunk. Sometimes these are the actions of a drunken person and sometimes a drunken animal such as a monkey. In the case of the fourth Dragon Dao Yin walk it is the movements of a drunken dragon we are trying to emulate; you may have to use your imagination to some degree for this!

Generally names are given to exercise and sequences in the Chinese arts in order to give a clue as to the essential feel of the movements we are trying to achieve. In Chinese medical thought alcohol is said to 'slacken' the Qi, as the Qi directing force of the Liver becomes compromised. This means that the energy flow of this exercise should be very relaxed and soft in order to reflect the soft Qi flow that is taking place in a drunken person. Any movement or style with the word 'drunken' in its name should also reflect this soft quality.

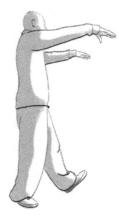

FIGURE 5.14: STARTING DRUNKARD WALKING

If you successfully managed the previous walking exercise then you should find the Drunkard Walking exercise simple in comparison. It uses much simpler body mechanics.

Begin from the position shown in Figure 5.14. Your weight is all back in your right leg whilst your left foot is in front. The heel of your front foot should be lightly touching the ground. Raise your arms lightly up in front of you and relax your wrists so that your hands and arms can fully relax. You should be in a somewhat 'zombie-like' posture. Just stand here for a few minutes and breathe normally. Let your body relax more and more so that your internal Qi flow can soften.

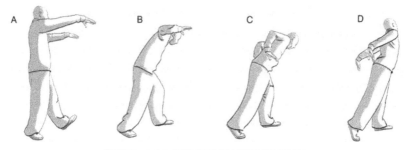

FIGURE 5.15: DRUNKARD WALKING (1)

Drunkard Walking is incredibly good for your body. It is especially good for opening up the line of the front of the body where many emotional pathogens stagnate. It opens up any collapse of the torso and clears stagnation from the region of the Heart.

Begin from your starting position, shown in image A of Figure 5.15, before shifting your weight forward into the front leg and slightly bringing your arms back to level with the top of your head, as shown in image B. Inhale as you do this.

Now stretch up your head into the sky and push back behind you with your palms. As you do this, stretch open the front of your body and press into the floor with the Yongquan (KI 1) point of the rear foot. Exhale strongly as you carry out this movement. This is shown in images C and D.

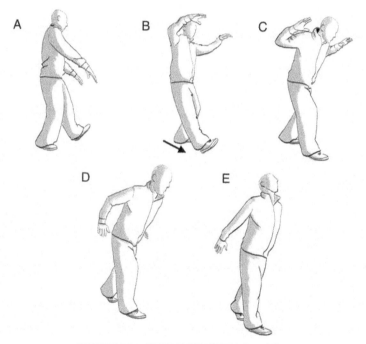

FIGURE 5.16: DRUNKARD WALKING (2)

Now we need to learn how to change direction with this walk and step forward. The previous exercises all took place in a straight line. Drunkard Walking is a little different as it emulates the disorientated stepping of an inebriated man/dragon. This means that the exercise 'zigzags' forward. Figure 5.16 shows exactly how we perform the change of direction and the second step of the Drunkard Walking exercise on the other side of the body.

Begin by rocking your weight back into the rear heel as shown in image A. Keep your body as relaxed as you can and lightly swing the arms forward so that they are in front of you. Begin to inhale as you do this.

Now rock around on your heels to face 45 degrees to your right. You should aim to rotate around your centreline and swing the body with a slightly 'drunk' feel. Now take a step forward with your rear foot as indicated by the arrow in image B.

Begin to exhale as you shift your weight forward into the front foot. Bring the arms back to level with the top of your head and then press them back as you extend your head and open your chest as shown in images C, D and E. This is the same movement you have already performed on the other side of the body.

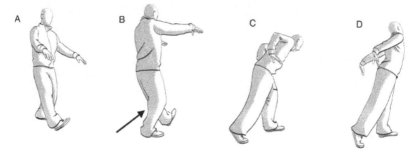

FIGURE 5.17: DRUNKARD WALKING (3)

Now repeat once more on the first side of the body. Shift your weight back as shown in image A as you swing your arms forward. Swing your body around 45 degrees to your left and take a step forward as shown in Figure 5.17, image B. You can now perform the stretch shown in images C and D once more.

Once you can successfully do this and string the movements together into a continuous walking exercise, you have learnt Drunkard Walking. As before, spend some time getting used to the exercise and then gradually begin to integrate the various Dao Yin principles from Chapter 4 of this book in order to bring the exercise to life.

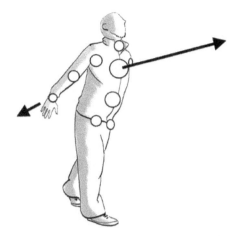

FIGURE 5.18: DRUNKARD WALKING QI MEN

Figure 5.18 shows the key Qi Men that are opened whilst performing this exercise. As you can see, they are mostly on the front of the body. It is a powerful stretching movement which also connects most of the Jing Jin pathways that run along the front of the body and arms. The two arrows shown in Figure 5.18 show where your Yi is extended. These arrows are included as the extension of Yi is a little different from before. In order to fully open the Qi Men around the Heart you should extend your intention out of the centre of the chest and at the same time backwards out of the palms, which are pushing behind you. This can be a little more complex than with the previous Dragon Dao Yin exercises as it is designed to set up a 'two-way' movement of energy that drags pathogens out from deep inside the body.

CONCLUDING THE FOUR DRAGON DAO YIN WALKS

These are the four complete Dragon Dao Yin walks which make up the beginner-level training contained in this book. Despite their foundational level they can actually be quite complex when you first start practising them, so be patient with yourself and persevere in order to ensure that you learn them correctly. Spend time integrating the various Dao Yin principles into them so that they begin to have some energetic functions as well as being a form of physical stretch. I would advise, when learning them, to work on one exercise at a time rather than trying to learn all four in one go. This is because each builds on the next.

For those who wish solely to improve their health and body posture there is no need to take these exercises any further than as outlined in this chapter. The four walks alone are more than adequate for learning how Dao Yin exercises work and for clearing much pathogenic energy out of the body. They have the advantage of taking you quite gently through this process whilst some of the more advanced practices are quite powerful in comparison.

For those who wish to explore the deeper aspects of Dao Yin training it is best to begin with the intermediate sequences taught in the next chapter before moving on to the advanced Dao Yin exercises explained towards the end of the book. These exercises are really for those wishing to move beyond the health aspects of the art into the more spiritual realms of Dao Yin training.

CHAPTER 6

Intermediate Practice
The Four Sequences

This chapter introduces the four full sequences of the Dragon Dao Yin exercises. These four short forms are based around the four walks that were discussed in Chapter 5. Learning the four Dragon Dao Yin sequences is more complex than simply learning the four walking Dao Yin which, it is advised, you should make sure you know before trying the exercises in this chapter.

Each sequence is introduced in turn, along with diagrams of the exercises being performed and information on what each exercise is aiming to achieve.

The four sequences are named as follows:

- The Awakening Dragon

- The Swimming Dragon

- The Soaring Dragon

- The Drunken Dragon

You will notice that each exercise begins and finishes in the same way, with the 'Circulating the Qi' exercise beginning the sequence whilst the 'Sinking the Qi' and 'Gathering the Qi' exercises conclude each form. These three exercises are actually Qi Gong rather than Dao Yin as they have the qualitative properties of Qi Gong exercises: the Yi is resting inside the body, there is no purging of pathogens and the Qi Men are not fully open. In this way each sequence mixes Qi Gong and Dao Yin methods into one form, ensuring the purging, nourishing and regulating of Qi takes place in each sequence.

Each sequence is also structured in a similar fashion. They each open with Qi Gong before you turn to the left and perform the walking exercises from Chapter 5. You then have a specific Dao Yin movement which turns you around on the spot before returning you to your starting position via a Dao Yin walk once more. Then the sequence brings you back to face forwards once again and closes with some simple Qi Gong. Each sequence is then concluded with a few minutes of standing, which is explored more in the Chapter 7.

DRAGON DAO YIN SEQUENCE 1: THE AWAKENING DRAGON

This is the first of the four Dragon Dao Yin sequences. It is based around the Piercing Palm walking exercise which you already know from studying Chapter 5. The name of the Dragon is more literally 'Waking up the Dragon' but this can cause confusion, as this term also refers to an advanced internal principle that I discuss in Chapter 7. In order to avoid any confusion I generally refer to this sequence as the 'Awakening Dragon'.

Figure 6.1 shows the starting posture for all four of the Dragon Dao Yin sequences.

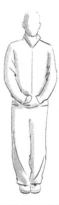

FIGURE 6.1: PREPARATORY POSTURE FOR THE DRAGON DAO YIN EXERCISES

Stand with your feet together and your knees slightly bent. Lightly close your eyes and rest your tongue on the roof of your mouth. Lightly clasp your hands in front of the lower abdomen and breathe naturally in and out through the nose. Note that the specific Dao Yin breathing method discussed in Chapter 4 of this book is not required for this posture, as it is a form of standing Qi Gong. You are not aiming to purge the energy body at this time. Remain in this position for a few minutes, try to relax your mind and empty it of thoughts. Rest your mind gently inside the lower abdomen where the lower Dan Tien is located.

The more effectively you can relax your mind and slow down your thoughts at this stage, the more effective the exercise will be. Preparation is everything in the internal arts, as moving mentally into this Yin state prevents confusing directions being given to the Qi. Remember that every thought you have directs your internal energy to some degree, so excessive mental activity will start to move Qi in a way that is not required for the exercise.

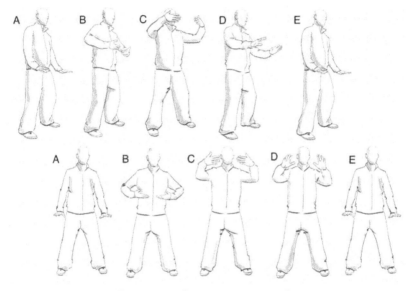

FIGURE 6.2: CIRCULATING THE QI

Figure 6.2 shows the first movement of the sequence. This is the Qi Gong exercise known as 'Circulating the Qi'. The exercise is shown from two different angles in order to help understand what the arms are doing.

Begin by stepping out from the previous posture with your left leg. Step out to a shoulders' width apart with the feet. Bring the hands to rest lightly in front of the hips with your palms facing the floor. Bend the knees slightly to take tension out of the legs. This should put you in the position shown in image A.

Inhale as you begin to raise the palms in front of you up to the height of your shoulders as shown in image B. Now begin to exhale as you extend the arms out in front of you in a circular fashion as if you are holding a beach ball; this is the position shown in image C, a posture often known as Zhuan Zhang or 'Standing Stake' in Qi Gong circles. From here continue to exhale as you bring the hands down in front of you as shown in images D and E. This should return you to your starting position for this exercise.

Perform this movement three times to begin the Awakening Dragon Dao Yin exercise. Note that standard abdominal breathing is fine for this exercise, as we are not trying to purge anything from the energy body right now. Let your mind lightly rest upon the lower Dan Tien and keep your eyes closed throughout this movement so that your mind is naturally led inside. The main function of this exercise is currently to ensure that Qi is being led through the meridians of the body and circulated effectively prior to purging any pathogens through the walking Dao Yin exercise. At an advanced stage in your practice the function of this exercise changes slightly and this is discussed in the next chapter.

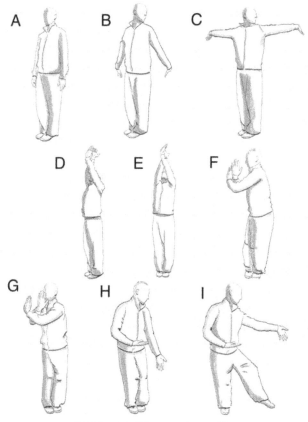

FIGURE 6.3: GREETING THE DAWN

Greeting the dawn enables us to move from our opening Qi Gong exercise into the first of our four Dao Yin walks. It helps to stretch open any Qi Men on the front of the body, as well as twisting our spine and lengthening along many of the Jing Jin lines of connective tissue. It is the first Dao

Yin movement of the sequence, and so we should now open our eyes and begin to switch our breathing method to Dao Yin breathing which encourages the purging process.

From the previous Qi Gong exercise step back in so that you are once more standing with your feet together. Any time we stand with our feet together in internal exercises, it is because it is then much easier to find the exact centre of our body. It is much easier for energy to focus itself towards the core of our meridian system. Relax your hands down; this should put you in the position shown in image A of Figure 6.3.

Now stretch open your chest as you turn over the hands and look to your left, as shown in image B. There should be quite a stretch on your chest and spine as you perform this movement. Begin to inhale at this point.

Lift the arms upwards whilst maintain a good stretch on the shoulders and chest as shown in image C.

Bring the arms in towards each other and cross the wrists as shown in images D and E. At this point you should twist around to the right, so that you have now twisted the spine to both the left and the right.

Sink into the legs and bring your arms down to your right, as shown in images F and G. At this point begin to exhale.

Swing the left arm past your body whilst keeping it fairly extended, as shown in image H. Keep swinging it past the body and exhaling whilst stepping out 90 degrees with the left leg and lightly touching the ground with the toes of your left foot. Your left arm wants to be quite extended at this point, with the Qi Men open and your left thumb extended into the distance. This is the position shown in image I. Your Yi should be extended far out into the distance as if you are trying to lead Qi out through the thumb of your left hand. This helps to begin purging the Lung meridian of pathogenic information, as the Lung meridian concludes on the end of your thumb. The right hand is lightly rested beneath the lower Dan Tien.

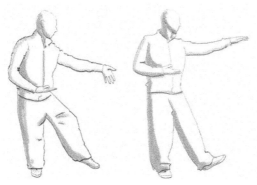

FIGURE 6.4: MOVING INTO THE WALK

Figure 6.4 shows a small transitional movement which often causes students confusion. It is not an exercise in its own right; rather it is just a method of moving from the previous exercise into the first of the four walks.

After hesitating for a short time in the previous posture, with your thumb extended, place your left heel down onto the floor and turn over your left hand so that it is now facing the floor. This will prepare you for the Piercing Palm walk.

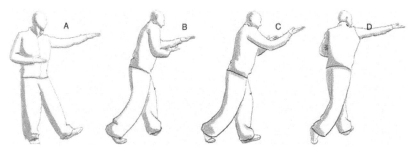

FIGURE 6.5: PIERCING PALM (1)

Now you are in the correct position from which to carry out the Piercing Palm walk from Chapter 5. If you have carried out the previous movement correctly you should now be facing 90 degrees to the left of your starting position, meaning that you will be walking to your left.

Carry out the first Piercing Palm step shown in Figure 6.5, as described in Chapter 5 (see pages 132–134).

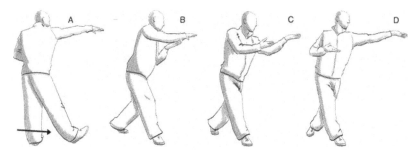

FIGURE 6.6: PIERCING PALM (2)

Now repeat the Piercing Palm exercise on the other side of your body as before, which constitutes the second step of the Dao Yin walk. This is shown in Figure 6.6.

Once you have done this you will have taken two steps. Repeat each step again so that you carry out four Dragon Dao Yin steps. This should leave you in the position shown in image D. You have now completed the first set of walking exercises in the Awakening Dragon sequence.

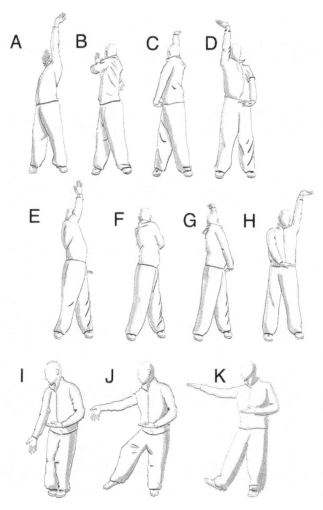

FIGURE 6.7: STRETCHING DRAGON (1)

You have walked to the left, and so we need a movement to turn ourselves around. This turning movement is called 'Stretching Dragon'. This move can at first seem a little complex but once you have tried it a few times you will find that it is actually quite simple.

From the previous position bring your left foot around to the front, as shown in image A of Figure 6.7. You will now have your weight evenly distributed between your feet, which will be facing in the same direction as you were facing when you began the sequence. Lift up your left arm high into the air and stretch out your right arm behind you. Now lift the right arm upwards as you lower your left arm. Keep stretching as much as you can throughout this movement. Keep going until they have switched and now the right arm is in the air and the left arm is stretched downwards. This is shown in images B and C.

Now, keeping the stretch on both arms, turn your body around to the left as shown in images D and E. Repeat the switching of the arms so that the right arm now moves downwards and the left arm moves upwards. This is shown in images F and G.

Once you have switched the arms around, turn your body around to the right, so that it returns to the front as shown in image H. This is all carried out quite quickly once you have a feel for the movement and should all happen on an inhalation. The combination of inhaling and working the arms in this way strengthens the Lungs, as the opening of the shoulders pulls on the origin of the Lung meridian which is on the outside of the chest near your shoulders. It also helps to start pulling pathogenic stagnation away from the chest towards your hands.

Begin to exhale as you swing the right hand out in front of you and step out with your right toes as shown in images I and J. This should put you back into a position you have already practised on the other side of your body (see Figure 6.4). Once more you should extend your Yi into the distance and stretch out the thumb.

Remain in the position shown in image J for a few seconds to allow the purging process to continue, before placing the heel down and turning your palm over as shown in image K.

This whole movement should form a powerful stretch which works the Lungs, the waist, the front of the body, the spine and the shoulders. Work on this exercise until it is natural and smooth with no obvious breaks in the twisting movements.

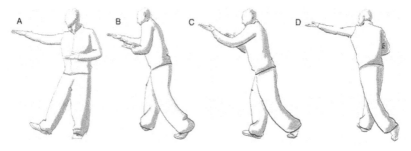

FIGURE 6.8: PIERCING PALM (3)

Twist on your right heel and extend out your left arm as shown in images A–D of Figure 6.8. You have now performed another step from the Piercing Palm, returning back towards where you started the sequence.

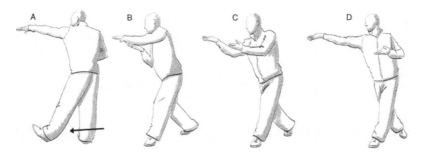

FIGURE 6.9: PIERCING PALM (4)

Carry out a second step of the Piercing Palm exercise as shown in Figure 6.9. This will mean you have completed two Piercing Palm steps. Repeat once on each side of the body so that you have taken four Piercing Palm steps, leaving you in the posture shown in image D of Figure 6.9. This is all of the Piercing Palm movements of the Awakening Dragon sequence completed.

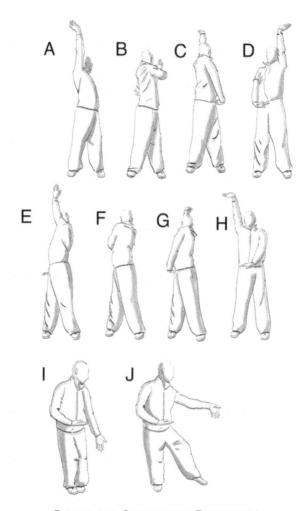

FIGURE 6.10: STRETCHING DRAGON (2)

Now step up with your rear leg and repeat the Stretching Dragon sequence as before, but this time on the opposite side of your body. This should take you through the sequence shown in Figure 6.10, images A–J. You should finish back on the spot you started the sequence from. If you are not, then something has gone wrong! Do not worry, try again and work through the images and instructions more slowly.

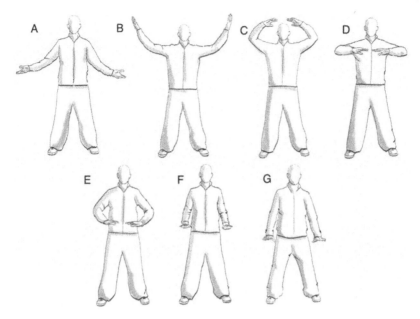

FIGURE 6.11: SINKING THE QI

Now bring your left foot around to the front once more with your feet a shoulders' width apart. This should leave you facing in the direction you began the Awakening Dragon sequence. Now we leave the Dao Yin aspect of the sequence and return to some concluding Qi Gong movements as shown in Figure 6.11. This movement is known as 'Sinking the Qi'. It is designed to bring any internal energy which has strongly moved during the act of purging back down in the body. This has calming effects upon the mind and the body, as well as ensuring that any excess energy can be move out into the planet where it is effectively 'earthed'.

Begin to lift your arms up over your head as shown in images A–C of Figure 6.11. You should inhale deeply and allow the speed of your breathing to dictate the speed of the entire movement. Exhale as you bring the arms in over your head and down the body in front of you, as shown in images D and E. As you bring your arms downwards you should gently bring your mind down through the centre of the body, level with your hands. Your Yi should make a soft pass through the body downwards as your hands move towards your hips. This pass of the mind helps any stuck Qi to move downwards into the planet.

As your hands reach the level of your hips they begin to rotate around to your sides as shown in image F. This means that your fingers are facing directly forwards. Now begin to push the hands downwards with a little force towards the floor. This helps to finally 'earth' any stuck Qi by utilising the power of a horizontally running meridian around your waist known as the 'girdling meridian'. This should put you in the position shown in image G.

Now repeat this movement twice more, so that you have performed the Sinking the Qi exercise three times.

On the last time through this movement hesitate at the position shown in image G. You should stay in this position for a few breaths and gently rest your mind beneath your palms as if you were quietly 'listening' to the space below your hands. This will help your Qi begin to move down towards the palms, ensuring that any Heat built up during the exercise is vented out through the palms via the Laogong (PC 8) meridian points.

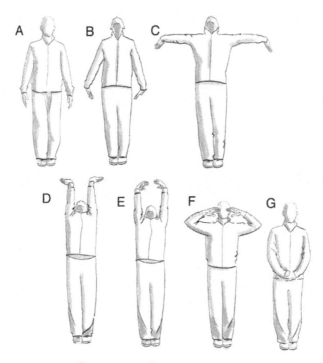

FIGURE 6.12: GATHERING THE QI

Figure 6.12 shows the final movement of the Awakening Dragon Dao Yin sequence. It is known as 'Gathering the Qi'. It is an unusual movement in that it is a characteristically Qi Gong exercise, but it is stretched out like a Dao Yin exercise. Its function is to finally connect the Jing Jin lines of the core of the body, stretch out the spine one last time and consolidate your Yi onto the lower Dan Tien.

Bring your left foot back in so that you are standing with your feet together. Relax your hands down by your sides. This should put you in the position shown in image A. Now roll open the chest and stretch open the heart area of your body as you look up towards the sky. This is shown in image B.

Lift the hands up above you whilst stretching open the shoulders and spine as shown in images C and D. Turn the hands over to face the floor whilst maintaining the stretch on your body. All of this from image A to E should be performed on an inhalation.

Now exhale and bring your hands down towards your lower Dan Tien. When you reach the lower Dan Tien relax your knees a little and lightly clasp the hands over the Dan Tien region of the body. At this point you should rest your mind on the lower Dan Tien, breathe long, slow, deep breaths in and out through the nose, and remain in this position for a few minutes. You have now completed the entire Awakening Dragon Dao Yin sequence.

Summary of the Awakening Dragon Sequence

In summary, the sequence of Awakening Dragon includes the following movements:

1. Standing in preparatory posture for a few minutes.

2. Circulating the Qi three times.

3. Greeting the Dawn.

4. Piercing Palm walk four times.

5. Stretching Dragon.

6. Piercing Palm walk four times.

7. Stretching Dragon.

8. Sinking the Qi.

9. Gathering the Qi.

10. Standing in closing posture.

DRAGON DAO YIN SEQUENCE 2:
THE SWIMMING DRAGON

The second of the four Dragon Dao Yin sequences is known as the 'Swimming Dragon'; it is based around the Dao Yin walking exercise from Chapter 5 called 'Dragon Plays with Pearl' (see pages 135–139). Within the internal arts world there are a number of exercises known as the Swimming Dragon exercise and they all look completely different. Some are based around sequences such as the Dao Yin form presented here, some are static postures and some involve complex coils of the spine. No matter what they look like externally, all of these exercises have one thing in common: they all work strongly to pump and cleanse the Kidneys. In alchemical texts the Kidneys are the physical manifestation of the element of water, which is why the dragon is said to be swimming, and the spine is always represented by the dragon. The health of the spine is dictated by the health of the Kidneys and almost all work with the Kidneys involves working the spine in some way.

The Swimming Dragon Dao Yin exercise begins in the same way as the previous sequence and follows the same structure: opening with Qi Gong, moving through some walking Dao Yin exercises which are directed to the left of your starting position, turning around using a Dao Yin exercise, and then returning to your starting position. The sequence then closes with the same Qi Gong exercises as the previous exercise as well. For many of the exercises, the details are the same as for the previous sequence. Where this is the case you should refer to the details from the Awakening Dragon sequence, but I have included the illustrations again here for convenience and ease of learning.

Figure 6.13 shows the preparatory posture for the Swimming Dragon exercise.

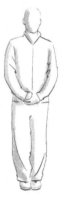

FIGURE 6.13: PREPARATORY POSTURE FOR SWIMMING DRAGON

Begin this sequence in the same way as the last with your mind relaxed, breathing deeply in and out through the nose. Rest your mind on the lower Dan Tien and prepare yourself for practice of the Swimming Dragon exercise.

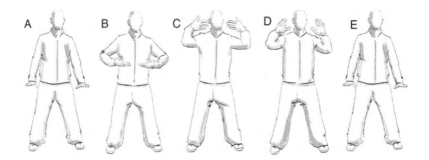

FIGURE 6.14: CIRCULATING THE QI

Figure 6.14 shows the Circulating the Qi exercise which opens the Swimming Dragon sequence. This is the same Qi Gong exercise as the one performed in the Awakening Dragon sequence and should be carried out with the same details in mind. This exercise opens each of the four Dao Yin sequences. You should repeat it three times before moving on to the next movement.

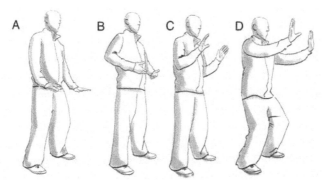

FIGURE 6.15: PUSHING THE TIDE

After finishing the previous posture, begin to sink down a little into your legs as you lift your hands up to your chest. At this point you should have your palms facing the sky and inhale as you begin the movement. This is shown in images A and B of Figure 6.15.

Exhale as you push your hands away from you as shown in images C and D. Extend your Yi out into the distance from both hands to help the purging process. As you do this, curve your lower back ever so slightly just to create a little more space for the physical organ of your kidneys. This will help any Cold pathogenic energy stuck around the area of the Kidneys to move out of the body via your palms.

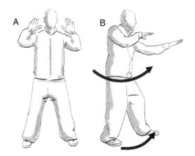

FIGURE 6.16: SWIMMING DRAGON TRANSITION

From the previous pushing posture pick up your left foot and step around to your left as shown in Figure 6.16. Allow your weight to drop into the centre with an equal weight distribution between both feet. Rotate your arms around with your body to the position shown in image B, which should prepare you to practise the Dragon Plays with Pearl walk. You should now be facing 90 degrees to the left of your starting position. This movement is carried out on an inhalation.

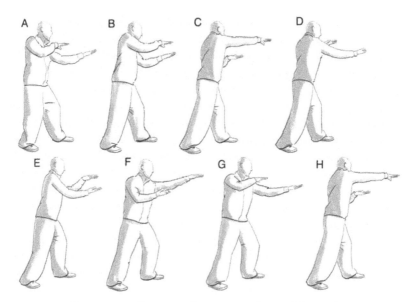

FIGURE 6.17: DRAGON PLAYS WITH PEARL WALK (1)

Now you are ready to perform the Dragon Plays with Pearl walk, which was discussed in the previous Chapter 5 (see pages 133–137). Carry it out in the same manner as shown in images A–H of Figure 6.17. Ensure that you have the correct breathing method, strong intention and all of the Dao Yin principles integrated into the movements.

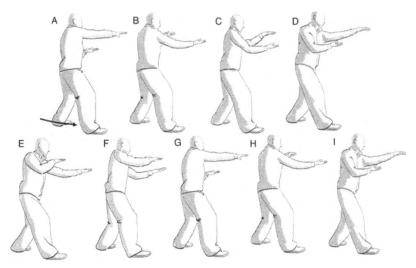

FIGURE 6.18: DRAGON PLAYS WITH PEARL WALK (2)

Now step through with your rear foot and carry out the Dragon plays with Pearl walk on the second side of your body, as shown in Figure 6.18, images A–I. You should now have completed two steps of the walking exercise.

Repeat these movements twice more for a total of four steps forward, so that you finish the four steps in the position shown in image I of Figure 6.18.

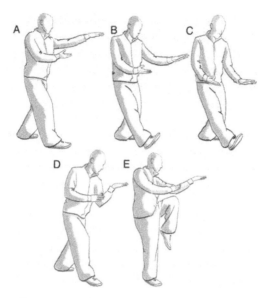

FIGURE 6.19: PRESENTING PALM TO HEAVEN

Presenting Palm to Heaven is probably the most difficult of the movements from the Swimming Dragon sequence. It is designed to help nourish the Kidneys and connect them in energetically to the Heart via the Chong Mai.

First rock your weight back into the rear foot whilst lifting the toes of your front foot, as shown in images B and C of Figure 6.19. Now shift your weight back into the front foot as you lift your left knee as high as you can into the air; you should now be standing on one leg, as shown in image E. The fingers of your right hand should lightly touch the inner elbow crease of the left hand, which is slightly extended with the palm facing the sky. The inner crease of your elbow is a powerful 'pooling' area for the Qi that flows through the Heart and Pericardium meridians; by lightly touching here we help stimulate the energy of these two organs.

Remain on one leg for a few breaths and stare out into the distance whilst extending your Yi out through the fingers of your front hand. By lifting the knee in this way we stretch the lower back to affect the Kidneys.

Inhalation during this exercise is carried out as we sink backwards, as in images A–C. Exhalation is through images D and E.

In many forms of internal exercise, when we stand on one leg we are causing a very fine central point of balance in the body. This helps to direct Qi in towards the centre of our body, leading it towards the central branch of the Chong Mai, which is discussed in more detail in Chapter 7. It is through this branch of the meridian system that the Kidneys and Heart internally communicate with each other and we are trying to assist in this process.

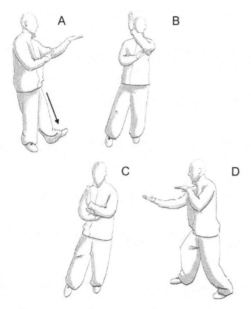

FIGURE 6.20: SWIMMING DRAGON TURN

From position E in Figure 6.19 place your left heel down onto the floor. Now shift your body around and transfer your weight into the left leg, as shown in image B. Bring your left arm around and bring it down in front of your heart to help affect the energy of the Chong Mai. Now step around with your right foot, as shown in Figure 6.20, image D. Relax your weight evenly between both feet and bring your right arm over to the position shown in D. This will have turned you 180 degrees, ready to begin the Swimming Dragon walk back in the opposite position.

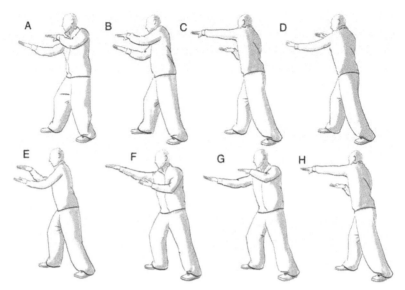

FIGURE 6.21: DRAGON PLAYS WITH PEARL WALK IN REVERSE (1)

You should now be facing back towards your starting position, as the previous two movements have rotated you around 180 degrees. Perform the Dragon Plays with Pearl walk again on this side of the body in exactly the same way.

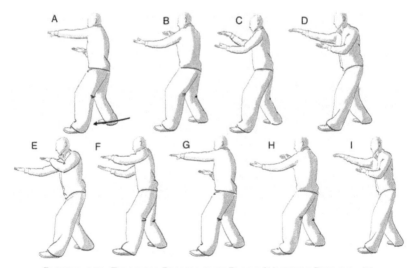

FIGURE 6.22: DRAGON PLAYS WITH PEARL WALK IN REVERSE (2)

Take a step forward as shown in Figure 6.22, image A and complete a second step of the Dragon Plays with Pearl walk on this side of the body. Once you have done this, repeat once more on each side of the body for a total of four steps. You have now completed all of the walking Dao Yin movements for this sequence.

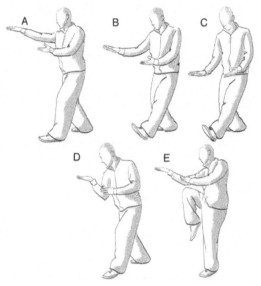

FIGURE 6.23: PRESENTING PALM TO HEAVEN

In order to turn around you should now carry out the Presenting Palm to Heaven exercise once more on the opposite side of the body, as shown in Figure 6.23. This can feel a little strange on this side of the body when you first start practising it but with a little perseverance it will start to feel natural. Make sure that all of the details discussed earlier are applied (see page 168).

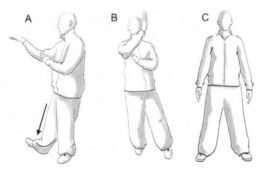

FIGURE 6.24: SWIMMING DRAGON TURN

Repeat the process of turning around as before. Follow the earlier directions (see page 169) and move through images A to C of Figure 6.24.

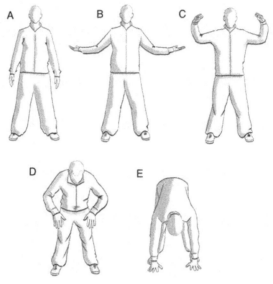

FIGURE 6.25: DIVING DRAGON

After completing the previous movement in Figure 6.24, you should be able to step lightly into the position shown in image A of Figure 6.25. Your feet are a shoulders' width apart and your hands are resting lightly at your sides. You should now be facing in the same direction as you were at the start of the sequence.

Inhale and begin to bring your arms up and over your head, as shown in images B and C. It can feel difficult at first, but try to lift the muscles of your back a little as you do this so that the area around the lower spine is opened. This helps to stimulate the Kidneys one last time as we complete the Swimming Dragon sequence.

Exhale as you lower your body down towards the floor, as shown in image D. If you can reach, bring your palms flat to the floor with your legs straight, as shown in image E. If you cannot reach the floor then relax and try to touch your toes with the tips of your fingers, although you should aim to build up towards touching your palms to the floor.

Extend your mind down a long way into the floor through your palms as you hold this position. Stay here and breathe for a while to allow any stuck pathogens around the lower spine to move through and out of your arms.

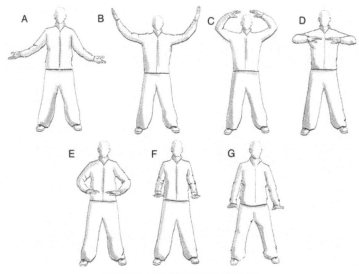

FIGURE 6.26: SINKING THE QI

As with the previous Dao Yin sequence, we finish the Swimming Dragon form by performing the Sinking the Qi exercise three times as shown in Figure 6.26. The details of the practice are exactly the same as for the Awakening Dragon sequence (see pages 161–162), including the hesitation of the hands at the height of the hips for a few breaths at the end of the third time through the movement.

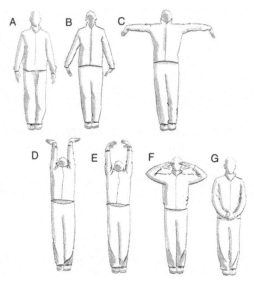

FIGURE 6.27: GATHERING THE QI

Figure 6.27 shows the Gathering the Qi movement which closes each of the four Dragon Dao Yin sequences. The details are the same as for the closing of the Awakening the Dragon sequence, so please refer back to pages 162–163 for instruction on this exercise.

As before, stand in the position shown in image G with your eyes closed for a few minutes, and breathe gently. Keep your mind rested lightly on the lower Dan Tien.

Summary of the Swimming Dragon Sequence

In summary, the sequence of the Swimming Dragon Dao Yin includes the following movements:

1. Standing in preparatory posture for a few minutes.
2. Circulating the Qi three times.
3. Pushing the Tide.
4. Dragon Plays with Pearl walk four times.
5. Presenting Palm to Heaven.
6. Swimming Dragon Turn.
7. Dragon Plays with Pearl walk four times.
8. Presenting Palm to Heaven.
9. Swimming Dragon Turn.
10. Diving Dragon.
11. Sinking the Qi.
12. Gathering the Qi.
13. Standing in closing posture.

DRAGON DAO YIN SEQUENCE 3:
THE SOARING DRAGON

The Soaring Dragon is the third of the Dragon Dao Yin sequences. It has fewer movements than the other three Dao Yin, but can be more challenging with regard to body mechanics and co-ordination. It is a very strong exercise for opening up the entire chest, upper back and neck area of the body so that tension is relieved and stagnation is purged.

This sequence is based around the Flying Dragon walk with which you will already be very familiar from Chapter 6. There is also the option of choosing a more physically demanding version of the Flying Dragon walk for those who want to fully work their legs and hips. This is optional though, and only recommended for those who are sure they have the required level of flexibility and body conditioning. If you push yourself beyond what is comfortable for the body you are likely to end up hurting yourself, so only progress onto the more challenging version of the Flying Dragon walk when you are sure you are ready.

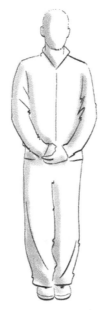

FIGURE 6.28: PREPARATORY POSTURE FOR SOARING DRAGON

As with the previous two sequences, the Soaring Dragon Dao Yin begins from the position shown in Figure 6.28. Remain here with your mind on the lower Dan Tien, breathing gently, before beginning the practice.

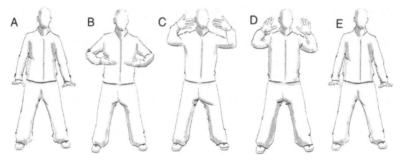

FIGURE 6.29: CIRCULATING THE QI

From the preparatory posture step out with your left foot to shoulders' width apart and begin the Qi Gong exercise known as Circulating the Qi, which is shown again for your convenience in Figure 6.29.

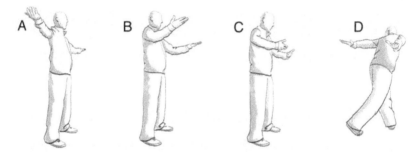

FIGURE 6.30: BEGINNING THE FLYING DRAGON WALK

Once you have performed the previous movement three times it is time to move into the first step of the Flying Dragon walk, as shown in Figure 6.30. As with the previous two sequences, you should perform this movement with a step out 90 degrees to your left. It is in this direction that you will perform the entire Flying Dragon walking sequence.

Raise your arms up to your sides as shown in image A. Keep them relaxed and have the feeling that they are floating up into the air by your sides. Inhale as you perform this movement.

Now bring your hands back towards your armpits with your palms facing the sky, as shown in images B and C.

Exhale as you take a small step with the left foot and rotate around your heel, twisting the entire body strongly around to the left. Look over your left shoulder to ensure that the cervical vertebrae are included in the twisting motion you are putting into the spine. As you do this, extend your hands out from beneath your armpits and stretch them out so that the joints in your chest, shoulders and arms are fully extended. This should put you in the posture shown in image D.

Note that although this is just a transition movement to get you from the opening Qi Gong of the sequence into the Dao Yin walking exercise, it also counts as the first of the four steps you are going to perform. It is important that you keep this in mind and recognise this movement as the first step, or you will end up facing in the wrong direction halfway through the sequence.

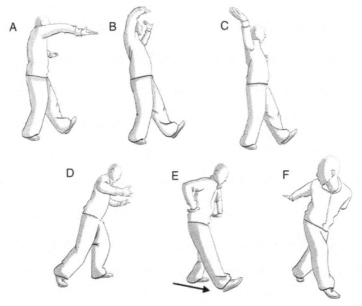

FIGURE 6.31: FLYING DRAGON WALK (1)

From the previous posture lean backwards and circle your arms around to above your head, as shown in images A and B of Figure 6.31. From here continue into the second step of the Flying Dragon walking exercise as discussed in Chapter 5 (see pages 143–144). You should already be familiar with this movement.

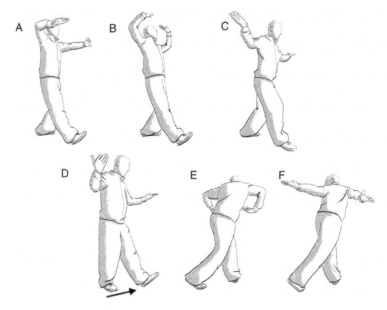

FIGURE 6.32: FLYING DRAGON WALK (2)

Perform the third step of the Flying Dragon walking exercise as shown in Figure 6.32. This is exactly the same movement as you have previously practised. This should conclude step three of the walking section of this sequence.

From here continue once more and complete a fourth step, which should place you in the position shown in image F of Figure 6.31. If you are in the same position as this, then well done, you have just successfully completed four steps of the Flying Dragon walking exercise. If you have made a mistake then do not worry, it can take some time to get this right as it is quite tricky. Be prepared to go back and work through the instructions a few times. When I was learning these exercises I found this particular movement very difficult.

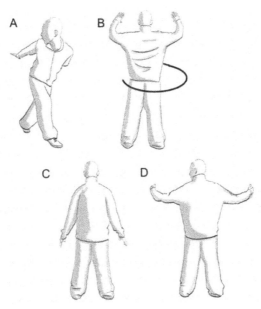

FIGURE 6.33: SOARING DRAGON TURN

From the previous position, which is shown in Figure 6.33, image A, rotate your body around to the rear. Your feet should stay on the spot whilst you do this; simply rotate around the heels. This is shown in image B. Lower your arms down to your sides as you exhale to bring them into the position shown in image C. Note that in the Soaring Dragon sequence you will be facing to the rear after completing the 'turnaround' posture, as opposed to facing in your starting position. Now raise your arms up to your sides once more and look to your left; this will prepare you for walking back in the opposite direction. This is shown in image D.

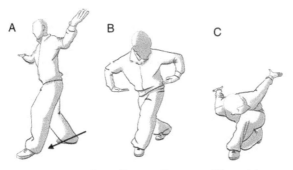

FIGURE 6.34: LOW FLYING DRAGON WALK (1)

At this point you have two options. You can either return back towards your starting position by repeating the Flying Dragon walk, or you can choose the more difficult option of performing the Low Flying Dragon walk, as shown in Figure 6.34. If you choose to stay with the high version of this posture then simply take four steps back to where you began the sequence, as described previously (see pages 176–177). If you select the more challenging option then follow the instructions below.

Begin by stepping out with your left foot as shown in image A of Figure 6.34. Raise your arms as if you are going to perform the high version of the Flying Dragon walk. Now, as you twist around to the left on your heel, begin to squat down a little. This is co-ordinated with the hands moving back in towards your armpits as before. Image B shows this movement.

At the culmination of this exercise you should fold down onto your right knee as shown in image C. Fully extend your arms backwards as you place your chest upon your knees, and exhale strongly. You should aim to fold the body up as much as you can when performing this exercise so that your hips and lower spine are worked as much as possible. In essence this is exactly the same as for the higher version of the Flying Dragon walk, it just adds a rotating squat at the completion of each step.

Please note that this walk can be very demanding upon the lower body. Only practise this movement if you are completely comfortable doing so. If there is any kind of pain in the hips or knees then immediately stop, and refrain from performing this exercise. It can take a long time to repair any damage you cause to the joints of your lower body by pushing yourself beyond your limits.

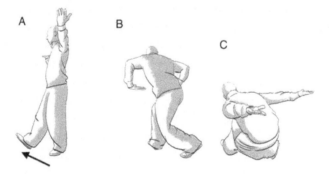

FIGURE 6.35: LOW FLYING DRAGON WALK (2)

So far you have completed one step of the low version of the Flying Dragon walk. Now continue and take step two, as shown in Figure 6.35.

Unfold from the joints of your hips to stand up and take a step forward with the right foot as shown in image A. This is when you begin to circle your arms upwards over your head and open the chest. Inhale as you do this.

Now fold down into the hips in the same way as you exhale, as shown in images B and C. This is exactly the same movement being performed on the other side of the body. This will mean you have completed two low Flying Dragon steps.

Repeat these movements to take steps three and four of the low Flying Dragon walk.

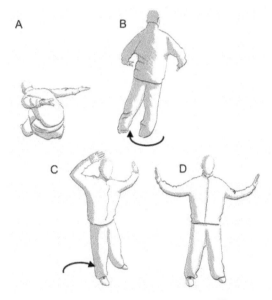

FIGURE 6.36: LOW FLYING DRAGON TURN

From the previous posture, which is shown in image A, Figure 6.36, you need to spin completely around to face the front. Raise yourself up and bring your left foot around in an arc whilst spinning on the ball of your right foot as shown in image B. This helps to stimulate the origin of the Kidney meridian on the base of your right foot. When you reach the front, step to a natural Qi Gong stance and exhale as you lower your hands down to your sides as shown in image D.

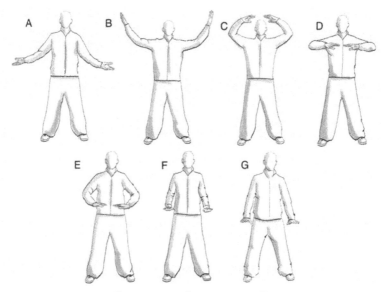

FIGURE 6.37: SINKING THE QI

As before, you should end up facing towards the front, as shown in image A of Figure 6.37. Now carry out the Sinking the Qi exercise as for the previous two sequences (see pages 161–162). Again carry out the movement three times, with a hesitation at the end of the third movement. This will help to settle the Qi down into the lower body and legs.

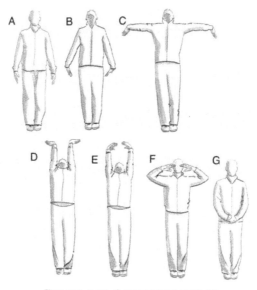

FIGURE 6.38: GATHERING THE QI

Figure 6.38 shows the Gathering the Qi exercise with which we finish all four of the Dragon Dao Yin sequences (see pages 162–163). As before, you should drop your awareness into the lower Dan Tien and breathe gently whilst standing for a few minutes to conclude your practice of the Soaring Dragon sequence.

Summary of the Soaring Dragon Sequence
In summary, the sequence of Soaring Dragon includes the following movements:

1. Standing in preparatory posture for a few minutes.

2. Circulating the Qi three times.

3. Flying Dragon walk four times.

4. Soaring Dragon Turn.

5. Low Flying Dragon walk four times.

6. Low Flying Dragon Turn.

7. Sinking the Qi.

8. Gathering the Qi.

9. Standing in closing posture.

DRAGON DAO YIN SEQUENCE 4: THE DRUNKEN DRAGON
The final Dragon Dao Yin exercise is the Drunken Dragon sequence, which is based around the Drunkard Walking movements that were discussed in detail in Chapter 5 (see pages 146–149). This is generally the last sequence that is practised during a session of working on the Dragon Dao Yin sequences, as it works through the length of the entire spine as well as helping to open the meridians which run along the spine's length.

As discussed earlier, any exercise which has the term 'drunken' in its name should be practised with a very soft feel to it. The Qi needs to be able to circulate without meeting any tension.

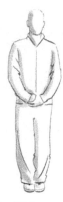

FIGURE 6.39: PREPARATORY POSTURE FOR DRUNKEN DRAGON

Begin the fourth Dragon Dao Yin sequence in the usual manner, in the posture shown in Figure 6.39, with your mind lightly resting upon the lower Dan Tien. Remain here for a few minutes, allow your mind to grow quiet and mentally prepare yourself for the practice of the following exercises.

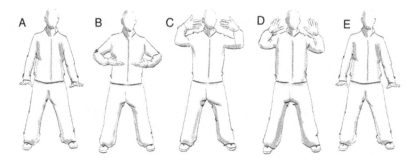

FIGURE 6.40: CIRCULATING THE QI

Perform the Circulating the Qi exercise shown in Figure 6.40 in the usual manner. Go through the movement three times in order to circulate your internal energy through the body in preparation for the coming Dao Yin movements.

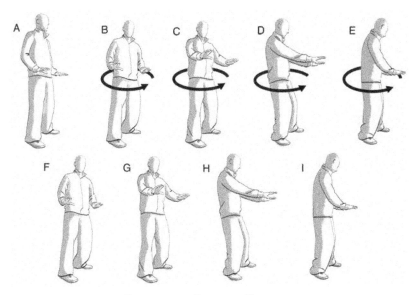

FIGURE 6.41: SWAYING DRAGON

The Swaying Dragon exercise shown in Figure 6.41 is an unusual movement designed to help the body locate its own energetic centre by swaying your body weight in circular movements. It engages a horizontally running meridian around your waist that helps to connect the lower Dan Tien into the rest of the energy body.

Begin in the posture shown in image A. This should be the position you are in after completing the opening Qi Gong exercise of the Drunken Dragon Dao Yin (see image E of Figure 6.40).

Keeping your feet still and without curving your spine, begin to sway backwards to your left as far as you can go without losing your balance. Now continue this movement into a circular swaying motion around your centre, as shown in images B to E of Figure 6.41. Follow the black arrow to ensure that you are swaying in the correct direction. Use your hands to help with maintaining your balance. Continue this swaying motion several times as shown in images F to I. There is no correct number of circles to make with this movement; four of five should be adequate to create the desired effects upon the energy body. Breathe normally throughout and do not worry about co-ordinating your breathing with the movements. Try to emulate the soft, swaying movements of a drunken person whilst performing this exercise.

When you have finished the movements, return to the neutral Qi Gong standing position shown in image A. This should still leave you facing in the same direction as when you started the movement, as your feet should not have moved.

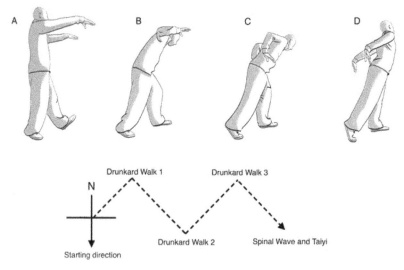

FIGURE 6.42: DRUNKARD WALKING (1)

Now you are going to move into the first walking section of the Drunken Dragon sequence. Once again you should move to your left, but this time the angle is larger. I have indicated the desired angle at which you should be facing in Figure 6.42. The chart beneath the images of the Drunkard Walking being performed is a very common way of representing the 'shape' of a form in Chinese instructional books. The compass chart is your reference point for your starting position. From here you should move into the first step of Drunkard Walking in the direction indicated, 45 degrees back to your left. Then the zigzag-style stepping is followed throughout the form until you reach the stage of turning around.

Turn to your rear left as shown in image A. Step out slightly with your left foot, raising your hands above your head as shown. Inhale at this point. Continue through the Drunkard Walking stretch as shown in images B–D, in the same manner as described in Chapter 5 (see pages 146–147). This is the first of your three Drunkard Walking steps.

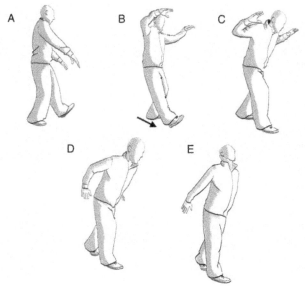

FIGURE 6.43: DRUNKARD WALKING (2)

Rotate in the direction shown in the chart and perform the second step of your Drunkard Walking, as shown in images A to E of Figure 6.43.

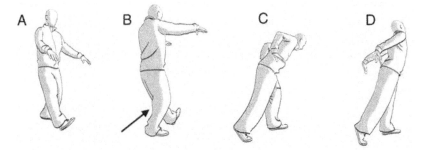

FIGURE 6.44: DRUNKARD WALKING (3)

Finish this section of the Drunken Dragon sequence by performing the third Drunkard Walking exercise as shown in Figure 6.44. This is the movement shown in images A through to D.

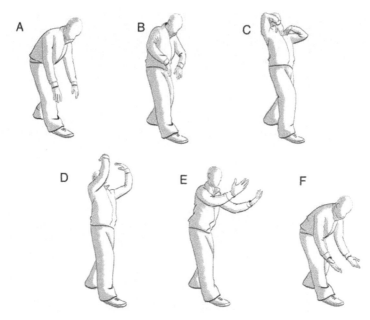

FIGURE 6.45: SPINAL WAVE

After completing three stages of Drunkard Walking you should move into the position shown in image A of Figure 6.45. Your right foot should have stepped forward into a small stance. Now relax your spine and arms and hang down with no power in the body other than a little strength in the abdominal muscles in order to stop yourself from fully collapsing to the floor. You should feel much like a marionette with your strings cut at this point. Your weight can rest evenly between your feet.

Begin to inhale as you send a soft wave up through the length of your spine. This should open each of the spaces between your vertebrae as you raise your arms as shown in images B, C and D.

Now exhale and relax your body forwards once more, with your arms performing a circling motion out from the body as shown in images E and F. This is one completed Spinal Wave exercise. You should repeat this movement three times without moving your feet in order to complete this section of the form.

This exercise opens up the entire length of the spine and relaxes all of the muscle of the back. The actual size of the movement will depend entirely upon your flexibility and core strength. Figure 6.45 shows a moderate level of spinal movement, but I have students who perform much smaller movements and others who really roll their spine in a very extravagant manner; either way is correct.

Early on in my school this exercise was dubbed the 'Drunk Dragon Vomits' due to the feel of the internal muscles moving during the exercise and the movement that the arms make. This name seems to have stuck and I am not sure if my students even remember that it was originally called the Spinal Wave! If you keep this somewhat distasteful image in your head whilst performing the exercise, though, you will start to get a feel of how it is supposed to be performed.

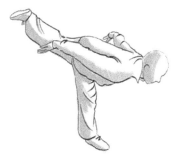

FIGURE 6.46: TAIYI STANDING

From the previous exercise tip yourself forward onto your front foot so that all of your body weight is on one leg. Lift the rear leg up into the air so that the base of your foot faces the sky and stretch open your chest as shown in Figure 6.46. Breathe naturally as you hold this position for a short while.

The term 'Taiyi' is a philosophical principle referring to a single point of focus. It is the 'one' produced from the nothingness of Wuji and the stage prior to the formation of Yin and Yang. For the purposes of the exercise Taiyi refers to the focus of the energy onto the Chong Mai, which is discussed in detail in the next chapter. As we lean forward and stretch open the chest we direct the force of the Chong Mai up into the Heart centre, helping it to open up. Medically, standing this way is also useful for the groin area and increases the health of the sexual organs, as well as being very good for your balance.

I never really understood how this movement fitted into the imagery of a drunken dragon until I taught the posture to a class full of people. I suddenly understood as I watched around 20 beginners hopping around on one leg, swaying from side to side and collapsing in a heap; they did indeed look drunk!

Take your time with this posture and work your way into this position. Do not overly push yourself or you will do your body some damage. It is okay to just tip your body ever so slightly forward when you first begin to practise this posture. As your confidence increases you can tip yourself further forward until you are in the full position.

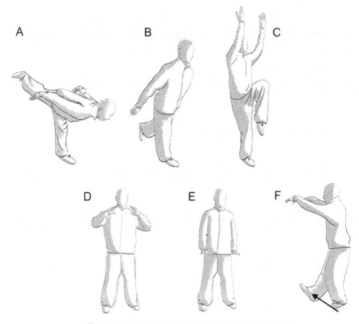

FIGURE 6.47: DRUNKEN DRAGON TURN

From the previous position of being balanced on one leg you should now move through the sequence of movement shown in images A–F of Figure 6.47. This will turn you completely around to face the opposite direction. From the one-legged posture lower your extended leg towards the ground, as shown in image B. Before your foot actually touches the floor you should bring it through in front of you and raise your knee as high as possible, along with your arms, as shown in image C. Your hands should twist inwards to help develop a strong feeling of torque through the upper limbs and torso. Now lower your foot to the floor until you are in a standard Qi Gong stance. Bring your arms down towards your hips as you exhale. This is the movement shown in images D and E. From here step around with your right foot to the rear and raise your arms upwards in front of you. This will put you in a position ready to begin drunkard walking once more.

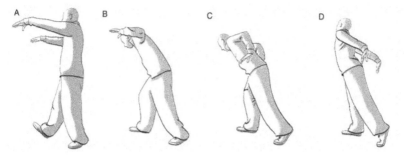

FIGURE 6.48: DRUNKARD WALKING (1)

From the previous exercise we simply rotate back around 45 degrees to our rear and perform the first of our Drunkard Walking steps, as shown in Figure 6.48.

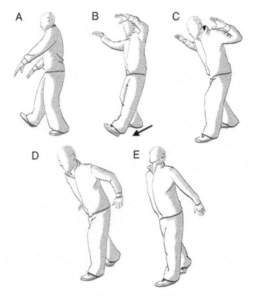

FIGURE 6.49: DRUNKARD WALKING (2)

Perform the second step of Drunkard Walking in the same manner as before. Your walking should be zigzagging you back to your starting position.

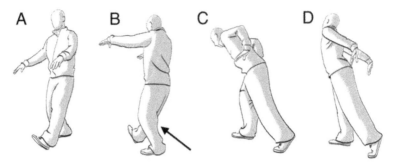

FIGURE 6.50: DRUNKARD WALKING (3)

The third step of Drunkard Walking, as shown in Figure 6.50, is the final part in the walking exercise section of this sequence. From here we can move back into the Spinal Wave exercise on the other side of the body.

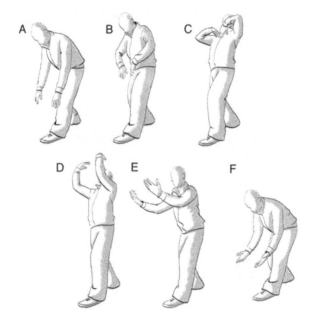

FIGURE 6.51: SPINAL WAVE

Carry out three repetitions of the Spinal Wave exercise as shown in Figure 6.51. The details for this movement are the same as described on page 188.

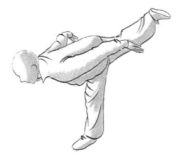

FIGURE 6.52: TAIYI STANDING

For the second time, lean forward and balance on one leg as shown in Figure 6.52. Hold this posture for a short while and breathe naturally.

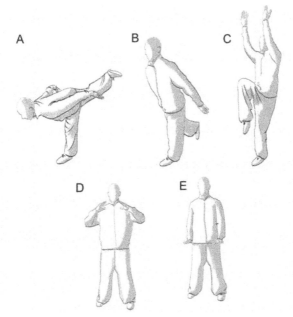

FIGURE 6.53: DRUNKEN DRAGON TURN

Repeat the process of turning around as before. This will take you through the process shown in images A–E of Figure 6.53. The only difference with this sequence is that instead of turning completely around, you finish facing the front, as shown in image E. This will put you into the correct position for the next movement.

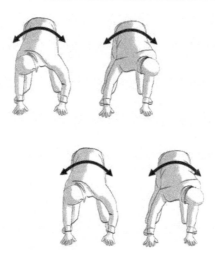

FIGURE 6.54: SPINE SHAKING

From the previous exercise lean forwards and place your hands on the floor as shown in Figure 6.54. If you cannot reach the floor then simply hang your body forwards as if trying to touch your toes, but you should aim to work towards fully reaching the ground. Extend your mind out through the palms, deep into the ground, to gain a solid energetic connection with the planet.

Now begin to shake your spine from side to side as shown in Figure 6.54. Fully shake open the spine and wiggle your hips whilst staying as relaxed as possible, to give your spine a last workout. Imagine the image of a dog and how it shakes the length of its body after getting out of a river. Try to emulate those smooth ripples it makes with its spine as it shakes.

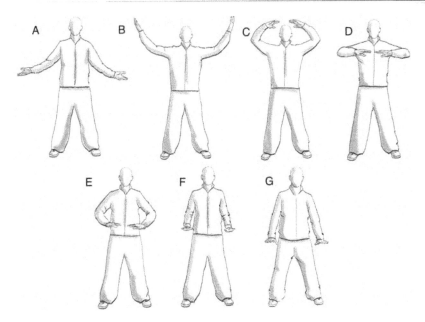

FIGURE 6.55: SINKING THE QI

Now we are moving on to the concluding Qi Gong exercises that make up the end of all four Dao Yin sequences. Carry out three of the Sinking the Qi movements as shown in Figure 6.55, images A–G. On the final repetition of the movement hesitate with the palms facing downwards by the sides of your hips. This will ensure that your Qi moves restfully down in the body if it needs to.

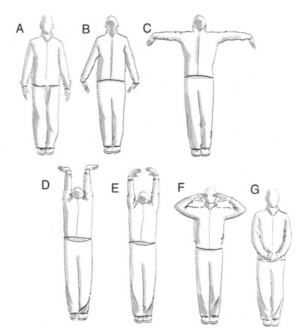

FIGURE 6.56: GATHERING THE QI

Close your Dragon Dao Yin practice by completing the Gathering the Qi movement as shown in Figure 6.56. Bring all of your awareness down into the lower Dan Tien and remain in the position depicted in image G. Remain here for a few minutes and breathe naturally. You have now completed the fourth Dragon Dao Yin sequence.

Summary of the Drunken Dragon Sequence

In summary, the sequence of the Drunken Dragon includes the following movements:

1. Standing in preparatory posture for a few minutes.

2. Circulating the Qi three times.

3. Swaying Dragon.

4. Drunkard Walking three times.

5. Spinal Wave.

6. Taiyi Standing.

7. Drunken Dragon Turn.

8. Drunkard Walking three times.

9. Spinal Wave.

10. Taiyi Standing.

11. Drunken Dragon Turn.

12. Spine Shaking.

13. Sinking the Qi three times.

14. Gathering the Qi.

15. Standing in closing posture.

These are the four Dragon Dao Yin sequences in their entirety. They may appear quite complex at first, but persevere and follow the instructions closely. It will not be long before you have the hang of the physical movements and then you can gradually implement all of the Dao Yin principles discussed in Chapter 4 into the exercises. From here you should spend some time getting to know the sequences and allowing your body to become familiar with the movements you are asking of it. Once you have maintained a regular, daily practice for some time, then it is time to begin moving on to the more advanced aspects of Dao Yin training discussed in the next chapter.

CHAPTER 7

ADVANCED PRACTICE
ENTER THE DRAGON

By this time you should be familiar with the four basic walks of the Dragon Dao Yin exercises as well as the short sequences that combine Qi Gong and Dao Yin training. These four short sequences are considered a more intermediate stage of training and they can take some time to learn, especially if you are not used to learning sequences of body movements. Those who also practise an art such as Taijiquan will be quite used to learning forms, so the Dragon Dao Yin sequences may not actually prove too difficult. However long it takes, do not worry. If you find learning sequences difficult then persevere, as this is an exercise in itself. Once you have managed to learn the four complete forms then you should find that learning sequences in the future is much easier.

Now it is time to look at the more advanced stages of training in the Dragon Dao Yin exercises, which paradoxically is also the most simple with regard to body movements. The rule in Daoism is that Yin and Yang are always transforming into each other. They circulate and switch back and forth in an endless cycle of stillness and movement. It is this change between the two poles of Yin and Yang that creates existence, and it is this principle that we wish to emulate in our training. According to Daoism, too much physical movement on its own is imbalanced and negative, and so is too much stillness. True harmony exists when the two come together.

The process of performing the Dragon Dao Yin moves from stillness or Yin when you stand and breathe before starting the exercises. From here we move into Yang as the movements are practised. After practising the movements we return to stillness as we stand once more. The advanced stage of training in the Dragon Dao Yin involves the awakening of the final Yang movements, which is sometimes known as 'Waking up the Dragon', 'Dragon Plays with Pearl' or sometimes 'Dragon Exits its Cave'. This is the final energetic movement of the Dragon Dao Yin exercises and one that transforms the exercises from being medical into spiritual in nature.

In order to reach this stage we must first have achieved two prior stages of development. The first is awakening of the lower Dan Tien and the next is the 'Merging of Kan and Li'. These are discussed below.

THE LOWER DAN TIEN

Situated in the lower abdomen is the largest of three energy centres known as the Dan Tien, which is usually translated as 'Elixir Fields'. Anybody beginning classical training in the internal arts, whether that be through sitting practice, Qi Gong or martial arts, will no doubt be familiar with the concept of the lower Dan Tien. The lower Dan Tien is a sphere of pure informational energy which sits in the lower abdomen below the level of the navel, directly above the perineum. Figure 7.1 shows its location.

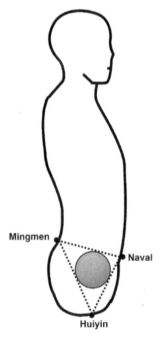

Mingmen

Naval

Huiyin

FIGURE 7.1: THE LOWER DAN TIEN

This sphere of energetic information is a part of the congenital energy body, which means that it is formed early on when we are in the womb. It carries out several key functions integral to our existence, which include the following:

- The lower Dan Tien converts our essence (Jing) into energetic information (Qi) throughout the course of our lives.

- The lower Dan Tien corresponds to an aspect of our thought processes, as intuitive thinking or 'gut feeling' is said to come from this area of the energy body.

- The lower Dan Tien rotates over a period of 24 hours, acting as a sort of 'driving wheel' that directs Qi through the meridians of the congenital energy body, which forms a cage of circulating energy in the body. This cage is shown in Figure 7.2. The movement of Qi in this cage then directs movement of Qi through the rest of the body's meridians giving us life. The circulations of Qi through the various parts of this cage are sometimes known as the 'small water wheels of Qi' or the 'microcosmic orbits'. Different Daoist schools of thought vary as to exactly how many of these circulations there are in the body.

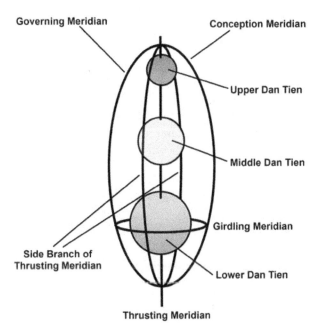

FIGURE 7.2: THE ENERGETIC CAGE OF THE CONGENITAL MERIDIANS

A key aspect of Daoist internal work from the spiritual tradition is the 'waking up' of this lower Dan Tien. This means that we increase its ability to rotate in order to increase the movement of Qi in the various 'small water wheels' of Qi in our congenital energy body. Those practising purely medical Qi Gong need not worry about this practice, as for purely medical purposes the lower Dan Tien need not rotate. The rotation we are aiming for mainly concerns those wishing to move from medical internal work into the realm of spiritual practice.

I have discussed the 'waking up' up of the lower Dan Tien in detail in my previous book, *Daoist Nei Gong: The Philosophical Art of Change*, and so will only discuss it here in brief, so as to avoid repetition. It is, however, necessary to understand in order to progress beyond the intermediate stages of training in the Dragon Dao Yin, so instruction is given here.

In order to wake up the lower Dan Tien we need three ingredients. These three are then combined alchemically in order to create the correct circumstances under which the Dan Tien will begin to awaken. The first ingredient is our breath, the second is the force of the planet and the third is our intention. If we only have one or two of these then the lower Dan Tien will remain dormant, but if we can bring all three together then the Dan Tien will begin to rotate more powerfully, which increases the energetic potential of our Dao Yin training.

LOWER DAN TIEN WORK

It is wise to wait until you are ready before you begin this kind of internal work. If a strong enough foundation is not built then the process will be more difficult. The stronger your prior foundation, the better. Generally it is advised that the following points are taken into consideration before progressing to direct work with the lower Dan Tien:

- You should have as open and relaxed a body as possible before working with the lower Dan Tien. It is advised that you only go on to this stage once you have practised Qi Gong, Dao Yin or something similar for some time already in order to build a strong bodily foundation.

- You need as smooth a flow of Qi around the body as possible in order to give the Dan Tien somewhere to direct the Qi flow as it rotates. Again, it is wise to have a good foundation in Daoist internal work prior to working on this stage. As a general rule I would advise several years of prior Qi Gong to build a good foundation. You could even use the Dragon Dao Yin exercises at the beginner and intermediate levels described in this book to build this foundation.

- Do not work on the lower Dan Tien when you are tired, as this will cause your essence to be affected.

- Do not combine this kind of work with drugs or alcohol. You want your body as clean as possible, so prepare for this work by abstaining from any toxic substances for several months before working with the lower Dan Tien.

- Do not engage in excessive sexual activity whilst working with the lower Dan Tien. As a general rule sex is fine as long as it does not leave you tired afterwards or with a weak back and legs. It is best to have a few weeks rest from sexual activity prior to beginning work with the lower Dan Tien.

- Never practise when there is any chance you may be pregnant, as the effects that it could have on a child are unknown to me. It may be fine, but since I always teach from personal experience I cannot verify this. I never teach any internal work to women who are pregnant as I feel that the energy is changing so fast for women at this time anyway that it does not seem sensible to then go and affect it even further through Nei Gong practice.

- Do not practise when you are feeling emotionally unstable. Wait for a time when you are feeling calm and relaxed before working with the lower Dan Tien.

You should have practised internal work for some time so you should be quite aware of the correct standing posture for working with the lower Dan Tien. All the standard postural rules from standard Qi Gong training apply. Adhering to these principles, stand in the posture shown in Figure 7.3.

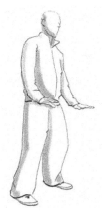

FIGURE 7.3: STANDING POSTURE FOR LOWER DAN TIEN WORK

Begin deep abdominal breathing, as discussed in Chapter 4 of this book (see pages 117–123). If you are familiar with the 'Sung Breathing' technique then feel free to use this instead. There is no need to use the 'Dao Yin Breathing' method from this book as we are not aiming to purge with this method. Ensure that your breath is smooth and even; make sure you expand the lower abdomen to the correct point, as discussed in Chapter 4 as this will cause the energetic pressure in the lower abdomen to stimulate the lower Dan Tien.

Now we wish to add the second ingredient – the force of the planet. This is a slightly different method from the one outlined in my previous book. There are several methods, each as effective as the next. I have found the version outlined here to be useful as many people connect with it quite easily when I am teaching.

The force of the planet reacts with our body throughout the course of our daily lives. It does so through the power of gravity and through our centre of gravity, which can be moved around our body depending upon our posture. The majority of people carry their centre of gravity high in their chest with little thought of its exact location. Whilst this is fine for walking around and carrying out daily activities, it is not what we want for internal work. Instead we use our body alignments to take the weight off our body and drop it down through into our feet. We then bend our knees in order to drop the centre of gravity down in our body. This is the main reason why any Qi Gong teacher will tell you to gently bend your knees when you join their class. In order to get the most from the force of the planet we wish to bend our knees to the most effective degree, such that the centre of gravity connects with our lower Dan Tien.

It is enough for beginners in Qi Gong simply to relax their legs and bend them. For advanced practitioners, though, we need to study every aspect of our structure, including this leg bend. There is a simple way to ensure that this is correctly done. First stand straight up with your feet together and your legs straight, as shown in Figure 7.4.

As you can see from Figure 7.4, your centre of gravity will be placed high in the chest. In the image I have marked where my centre of gravity is when I stand like this but it will vary from person to person, depending upon your height and body shape. Now tune in to your body and feel where that centre of gravity is. This is easiest done with the eyes closed, and if you wish to make it clearer you can rock gently from side to side, as you should be able to feel the centre of gravity move as you lean from left to right.

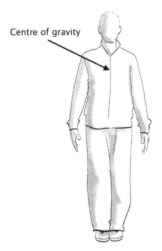

Centre of gravity

FIGURE 7.4: STANDING STRAIGHT

Once you have a feel for where your centre of gravity is, you wish to drop it down into the lower abdomen. Separate your feet and go back into the normal Qi Gong standing position. Gently bend your legs and sink down whilst tuning in to the point where your centre of gravity is focused. It should sink down in your body as you bend your knees. It is vitally important that we lead this centre of gravity down in the body until it lands directly on the location of the lower Dan Tien. Figure 7.5 shows this principle.

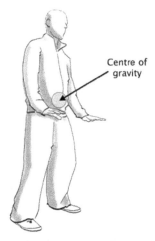

Centre of gravity

FIGURE 7.5: CENTRE ON THE LOWER DAN TIEN

The more exact you can make this location, the better. If you are quite internally aware then you will know when this happens, as your lower Dan Tien will heat up a little after around ten seconds of the centre of gravity coinciding with it. This is because the increased power of the planet reacting with the lower Dan Tien is stimulating the movement of essence in this area of the body.

It is wise to play with this and be very self-analytical. It can take a long time to get the exact location of the centre of gravity directly onto the lower Dan Tien, so keep checking and rechecking to make sure it is right.

In order to create space for the force of the planet to move up our body into the centre of gravity we need to ensure that we direct our body weight down into the Yongquan (KI 1) points on the base of the feet, which are shown in Figure 7.6. Ensure though that your heels are still on the floor. It should just be enough to direct your body weight forward until you feel the pressure move to the correct point. This means you will be making a very subtle shift forwards which is almost invisible to an onlooker.

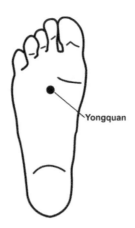

FIGURE 7.6: THE YONGQUAN (KI 1) POINTS

This enables more energy to be drawn up into the body. If the lower Dan Tien and the centre of gravity can coincide and you have shifted your weight to the correct point, then it will not be long before you begin to feel the vibration of the Qi of the Earth moving up your legs. This can make your legs shake a great deal, so do not worry; it is quite normal. This vibrating will gradually move up your legs until it reaches the lower abdomen, specifically the lower Dan Tien region. Your body temperature will go up, especially in your abdomen, and it is very normal to sweat.

Now we wish to add the third ingredient – your intention. Your Yi needs first to rest directly upon the lower Dan Tien. Now it needs to gently rotate the lower Dan Tien in the direction shown in Figure 7.7.

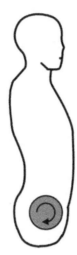

FIGURE 7.7: ROTATIONAL DIRECTION

Start slowly and get used to resting your awareness in the lower Dan Tien whilst it gently makes this forward turn. It is easiest to co-ordinate the turning with your breath so that the inhalation is the first half of the rotation, up the back of the lower Dan Tien, and the exhalation is the second half of the rotation, down the front of the lower Dan Tien. Stay with it and gradually the lower Dan Tien will begin to rotate. This will feel as though there is an actual sphere turning in your belly. It is very tangible and not something you could put down to just imagination, so keep going until the experience is strong. Do not be surprised if you get very hot and sweat profusely at this time.

The lower Dan Tien is directed in its rotation by the congenital meridians which surround it, and tethered to a central axis by four internal meridian points which appear as four yellow-coloured lights when you are able to see what is going on inside the body through the skill of 'inner vision'. These points have yellow lines extending from them into the middle of the Dan Tien and they can tug on the Dan Tien a little when it first wakes up. With time these four yellow cords disappear and the Dan Tien can spin freely, but this takes several years. When the cords tug on the lower Dan Tien it causes a slight lurch in its rotation which can cause the lower abdomen to react. It will twist spontaneously to one side and can even give quite violent jerks in either direction. Do not worry about this, even if it throws you off balance, it is all part of the process of waking up the Dan Tien; enjoy it!

The process of working with the lower Dan Tien in this way is an important part of Daoist Nei Gong training, and from here there are many practices and experiences to be had. Whilst this is a fascinating aspect of internal training it is not required for Dao Yin training, so it will not be explored here. Once the Dan Tien has even a little movement in it, even if it is not smooth, it is adequate for advanced Dao Yin practice.

THE MERGING OF KAN AND LI

Many times in Daoist literature you will hear the terms 'reversing Fire and Water', 'inverting Kan and Li' or 'merging Kan and Li'. These can cause confusion due to the symbolic language used in classical alchemical texts, but in essence all of these practices are quite simple, and often advanced practitioners will find that they begin to move into these stages automatically. All three of the above terms are referring to different practices and should not be confused with each other. For Dao Yin training we are only concerned with the 'merging of Kan and Li'.

Kan and Li are the names for two symbols in the *Yi Jing* (*Classic of Change*), an ancient text which discusses divination and the nature of energetic movement in the macrocosm. Kan and Li are often known as the Water and Fire Trigrams respectively and they appear as shown in Figure 7.8.

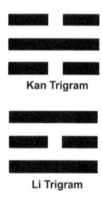

Kan Trigram

Li Trigram

FIGURE 7.8: THE KAN AND LI TRIGRAMS

The trigrams of the *Yi Jing* have multiple correspondences in the wider environment, in the human mind and also in the body. Internally they correspond to the organs of the Kidneys and the Heart , which are physical manifestations of the elements of Water and Fire. The Kan trigram, which is the Li trigram's opposite, represents the Kidneys. This symbol has two broken Yin lines enclosing a solid Yang line at the centre. Although the Kidneys' ultimate state is one of stillness, they must have the potential of Yang, a spark in their core, to function properly. The stillness of the Kidneys is said to be like a deep underground lake which holds the reserves of the body's essence, whilst the spark of Yang is known as the Ming Fire. This is an expansive ball of energy which sits on the base of the spine underneath the second lumbar vertebra. Its function is to generate warmth in the Kidneys, which helps to drive the essence out into the rest of the energy system. The Li trigram, which has two solid Yang lines moving outwards from the centre with a broken Yin line in the middle, represents the Heart. This represents the expanding movement of Qi which comes out from the Heart, and the ultimate stillness which sits at the Heart's centre. It is in the central hollow that the spirit of the Shen resides.

These two trigrams represent not just metaphysical concepts but also literal energies which reside in these areas of the body. They are two forms of Qi, which is essentially information. When the classics talk of merging the energies of Kan and Li they are referring to the practice of bringing the two energies together in the body to generate a reaction. This reaction is a mix of the two symbols which helps to create a new movement in the body. The new movement is created by the two poles of Yin and Yang dividing as Kan and Li are stimulated. This helps to create a greater degree of potential movement and the Chong Mai begins to open. This process is shown in Figure 7.9.

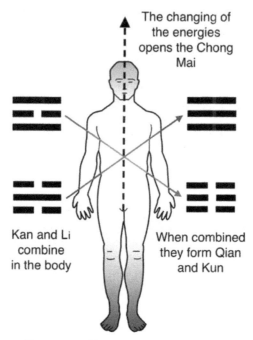

The changing of
the energies
opens the Chong
Mai

Kan and Li
combine
in the body

When combined
they form Qian
and Kun

FIGURE 7.9: MERGING OF KAN AND LI

Once the Chong Mai is opened up through this process, it connects into the awakened lower Dan Tien, and so we achieve the full energetic potential of the Dragon Dao Yin: the stage known as 'Waking up the Dragon'.

PRACTISING THE MERGING OF KAN AND LI

There are several different ways to merge the energies of Kan and Li. Some are from the alchemical tradition and involve sitting, whilst others are from the Qi Gong tradition and usually involve standing upright. It is from this tradition that we are going to take our exercise.

For this practice we are going to take the opening exercise of the four Dragon Dao Yin intermediate sequences. This is the simple Qi Gong practice which has already been discussed in detail in Chapter 6. It is shown again for convenience in Figure 7.10.

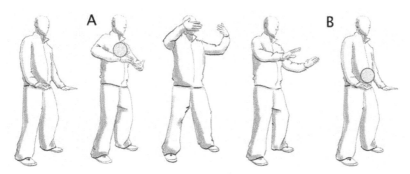

FIGURE 7.10: THE MERGING OF KAN AND LI EXERCISE

This exercise should be preformed in exactly the same manner as before, with a simple addition which will begin to engage the energies of Kan and Li. We do this by training a very acute awareness of the location of our centre of gravity whilst we are moving. In Figure 7.10 two postures are marked with letter A and letter B. A corresponds to the point where we have connected the force of the planet to the Heart's energy, and B corresponds to the connection of the planet's force to the energy of the Kidneys.

In the same way as we connected the planet's force to the lower Dan Tien in order to help it wake up, we can use this force to activate the power of the Kan and Li trigrams.

Carry out the exercise very slowly and try to focus on where your centre of gravity is within your body. When you come up into the posture marked as point A in Figure 7.10 you should aim to get the centre of gravity to sit right on the level of your Heart in the centre of your chest; this will actually be the location of your middle Dan Tien. As you exhale and sink down, lead that centre of gravity down into the lower abdomen, back into the lower Dan Tien, which is closely connected to the energy of the Kidneys and the conversion of essence which is stored in them. The skill with this to ensure that you make your control of the centre of gravity as accurate as possible. Be patient and spend some time ensuring that you are able to do this quite successfully. If you rush this stage then you will not build the required foundation for the next stage of development.

When you are starting to get comfortable with this you can begin to hesitate at these two postures for just a few breaths until you gain a strong feel for the movement of the planet's force through the body. If you have managed to attain this stage then you should become aware of a high-frequency vibration moving up the legs and through the body into each of the two energy centres in turn. This vibration will hit the lower Dan Tien as before, but now it will also reach up into the middle Dan Tien, causing your entire torso to vibrate. It can make you shake quite visibly sometimes and, as before, your body will sweat profusely as it begins to clear out toxins stored in the surface layers of the meridian system.

What you will notice is that carrying out this exercise shows you exactly what height you should be at when you practise Qi Gong exercises. In many systems of Qi Gong you straighten and bend the legs to move up and down, normally as you perform different movements with your arms. If you can co-ordinate the connection of the planet's force with your middle and lower Dan Tien then you will see exactly how much your legs need to fold and unfold. When you have gone beyond the beginner stages in your Qi Gong training this principle should apply to every movement that you carry out.

Now try adding this principle into the closing exercise of the intermediate Dragon Dao Yin sequences. This is the exercise shown in Figure 7.11.

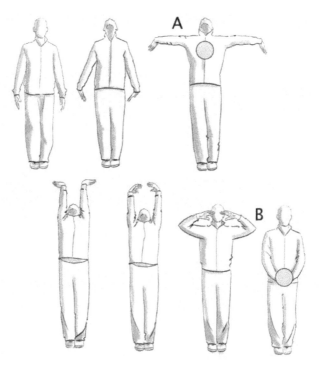

FIGURE 7.11: CLOSING WITH KAN AND LI

Again, A indicates the middle Dan Tien and B indicates the lower Dan Tien. When you finish this exercise you should move into the standing posture that concludes the Dragon Dao Yin exercises, with the planet's force directed towards the lower Dan Tien. Breathe naturally and bring your Yi to rest gently on the lower Dan Tien. Empty your mind as much as possible and just 'listen' to the lower Dan Tien for roughly ten minutes or so, without trying to do anything to it.

The first stage of learning any exercise is just to explore it, make sure that the principles are correct and try to get a feel for what is supposed to be happening. Apply this process to the above two exercises and try to gain an experiential understanding of connecting with the Kan and Li points. Once you have managed to do this you should then try to apply this to the practice of the four Dragon Dao Yin sequences. This means that you practise them as before with the principles of Dao Yin training throughout, but this time you also add the 'merging of Kan and Li' practice into the beginning and end of each sequence, as well as a few minutes' quiet standing. This is the basic process for 'Waking up the Dragon'.

THE CHONG MAI

The Chong Mai is often known as the 'thrusting meridian' or sometimes the 'central channel'. It is a long vertical pathway of energetic information which runs through the core of the congenital energy body. It is actually made up of several branches which are shown in Figure 7.12.

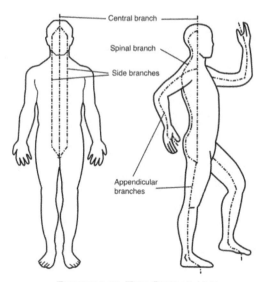

FIGURE 7.12: THE CHONG MAI

214 THE FOUR DRAGONS

The first branch is the straight vertical branch which runs directly through the core and connects the three Dan Tien together. It can be thought of as much like the pole that runs through a carousel horse. This is the key branch of the Chong Mai that is accessed and used in alchemical practices whereby Jing is transformed into Qi and then further into Shen. This is the process of lifting pure consciousness up into the upper Dan Tien in Daoist meditation practices. On either side of this central branch are two side channels which run through the torso. These assist in the alchemical process as well as governing the spiritual energies of the Liver and Spleen; they are very difficult channels to open and take quite some time. The rear branch of the Chong Mai system runs through the centre of the spine and it is this branch that we are primarily concerned with in Dao Yin training. The spinal branch is closely connected to the health of the mind and our thought processes, as well as our brain and its relationship to the nervous system. Clearing out the spinal branch of the Chong Mai greatly improves the state of our mind by assisting with the process of dissolving the acquired mind, which is discussed in Chapter 8.

It is within the spinal branch of the Chong Mai that the energy of the dragon is said to reside. Many forms of Qi Gong, Dao Yin and martial arts have postures and exercises named after a dragon. It is not always 100 per cent applicable, but in the majority of cases exercises with the term 'dragon' in their name usually involve a twisting or stretching of the spine. As the spine is manipulated, the branch of the Chong Mai which runs through the spine is accessed.

THE CHINESE DRAGON

To the ancient Chinese the dragon was a symbol of power and wisdom. It was a holy and venerated creature associated with spiritual growth; even today you will find dragon imagery all over China. With regard to the internal arts, the dragon symbolised a very specific process involving the transmuting of spiritual energy along the length of the spine and connecting this energy into the Dan Tien energy centres. It is for this reason that you will often see the same sort of dragon imagery repeated in classical Daoist artwork, paintings and carvings. The ancient Daoists outlined the alchemical processes of their study through the use of imagery. Figure 7.13 shows an example of this artwork taken from an old scroll.

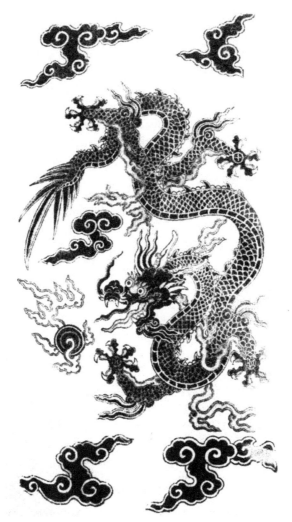

FIGURE 7.13: DRAGON CHASING THE PEARL

This is a very commonly depicted image of the dragon flying through the clouds chasing a flaming pearl, its body undulating and coiling as it moves through the air. Almost every Daoist temple complex I have ever visited had this symbol painted somewhere within its walls and this was the same in Tibet, Taiwan and many parts of southeast Asia. The picture of the dragon chasing the pearl depicts the process we are aiming to achieve through advanced practice of exercises such as the Dragon Dao Yin sequences.

The pearl in the image represents the lower Dan Tien. In alchemical traditions they would sometimes suggest that this actually showed the alchemical pill being formed within the consciousness, but I disagree. The pearl is generally flaming, which represents the heat of the lower abdomen as the essence begins to stir through our practice. This heat is clear to feel when the lower Dan Tien begins to awaken. In some Daoist dragon paintings you will see the dragon holding a smaller pearl between its claws, and this is the alchemical pill of Daoist meditation. The larger pearl being chased is the lower Dan Tien, and as such this particular image shows an earlier stage of development still working with the lower energy centre.

The body of the dragon is the movement of Qi along the length of the spinal branch of the Chong Mai. This energy spirals and twists its way through our back as the dragon awakens. The clouds which the dragon is flying through represent the Shen, our spiritual energy, which is increased by the movement of Qi up our spine. Shen is often depicted as clouds in order to demonstrate its ethereal nature.

So what does this mean? It is very important for me as a teacher that every single process inherent within the Daoist arts is very tangible. I feel that it is a great shame in the internal arts that so many processes and descriptions of processes are so vague. It is my experience that everything that happens to a diligent practitioner of the Daoist arts is very strong and clear to experience. This is the same for the movement of Qi along the length of the spine as the lower Dan Tien rotates, Kan and Li merge and our dormant dragon energy 'wakes up'.

In order to begin this process, finish performing one of the Dragon Dao Yin sequences, including the more advanced practices from within this chapter. Now bring your feet together and rest the mind on the lower Dan Tien as before. If you reached the right stage and built a solid enough foundation then it should be enough just to rest your mind on the lower Dan Tien, the driving force, and wait for the movement of energy to begin along the length of the spine. If it has not started after around ten minutes then it is still too early for you, do not worry, you need more time and practice.

When the energy moves along your spine, it spirals like the dragon in the painting. This causes your spine to spontaneously start moving. It will coil, stretch, undulate, twist and spring around inside your torso as if it has a life of its own. As this happens the Dan Tien will spin very quickly of its own accord and so your body temperature will rise. Do not be surprised if your body begins to jump around and you fall to the floor, it is all part of the process. Figure 7.14 shows a photo of one of my students experiencing this energetic phenomenon taking place in his body. As you can see, it produces fairly unsubtle movements.

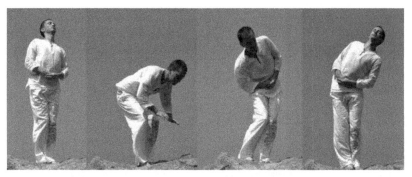

FIGURE 7.14: WAKING UP THE DRAGON

This reaction is caused by the Qi suddenly moving along the inside of your spine, which in turn causes the nervous system to react. It is causing the Chong Mai to open up and Qi movement to increase along the line of this meridian. It is also quite common to see a soft white glow in your head, if you do this with your eyes closed, as the Shen rises up into the upper Dan Tien. The clouds in the dragon painting indicate this.

This process can last from half an hour to an hour, depending upon what stage you have reached and what sort of state your internal energy system is in. It will subside naturally on its own. If you wish it to stop then simply separate your feet, breathe calmly, take the mind off the lower Dan Tien and then walk briskly around the room for a few minutes. It is quite normal to feel quite tired the first few times you experience this, and do not be surprised if you have slightly loose bowels after the first couple of these experiences. Think of it as a kind of internal colonic cleansing as the movement of energy attempts to clear stagnant toxins from the large intestine. The only major safety consideration to take into account is the fact that some of these movements are quite large. They can move you around a room with quite some force and sometimes with a lot of speed. This means that you should avoid having any sharp objects or corners around you when you practise. Make sure that your room is safe and spacious so that you are at no risk whatsoever.

This process is quite similar to spontaneous Kriya yoga practices, and indeed almost every spiritual tradition from the East discusses this taking place at some point. It is just a sign of the Chong Mai opening up and nothing to worry about. If you engage with this practice then you will notice that it goes through various stages and shifts. Sometimes it will be strong whilst other days it will be soft. The closer you are to a full moon, the more powerful the reaction will be. Once you have practised this for a while you will notice that the reaction gets much softer and almost vanishes altogether. At this stage you will just become aware of a gentle pulse along the length of the spine that an onlooker would most likely not even notice. When this stage is reached the spinal branch of the Chong Mai is opened.

THE FOUR DRAGONS

The Dragon exercises work on several different levels, depending upon how long you have practised them and how well you have integrated their principles into your energetic system. In general these are different stages I see people go through when I teach the four Dragon Dao Yin sequences:

- At first they are confusing and clumsy as you try to get the movements correct. This is the stage of tripping over your own feet, tightness in the muscles and much confusion. Do not worry when you are at this stage, everybody has to go through it and it will not last long!

- Once the sequences have been learnt and refined there is a stage where they feel just like stretches. They become almost like moving versions of the asana training from yoga. The exercises will feel internally quite empty but physically quite strong as they twist and pull your body into different shapes. They will cause your structure to realign, your joints to open and your posture to improve. This is an important stage and for many people the greatest boon to their health.

- After this you will begin to feel the body relax and the joints open and close as you perform the movements. This is the stage where the Qi Men begin to open up and the Jing Jin lines begin to connect together. The result is a feeling like elastic along the length of your body. This will improve your core strength, your connectivity, your flexibility and your balance.

- Usually it is after this that most students manage to integrate successfully the various internal principles of Dao Yin training into the movements. Now the Qi begins to move and the clearing process begins. Stagnant Qi is led from the body and the internal mechanics of the Dragon Dao Yin exercises can be experienced.

- The next stage involves the process discussed in this chapter. It is usually now that the Kan and Li merging practice can be applied to the sequences, and the energy of the spine begins to move. This is an advanced stage of training in the four Dragon Dao Yin forms.

- After some time at this stage you will begin to experience the differences between the four Dragon Dao Yin sequences with regard to how they affect the movement of Qi in your spine. Basically what happens is that each of the four forms sets up a different set of circumstances in your energy body. Different Qi Men are opened up and different Jing Jin lines are stretched open. Doing this causes a different quality of spinal energy movement when you enter the standing practice at the end of the sequence. These movements will be different from person to person and with time you will discover which of the Dragon Dao Yin forms is the most beneficial for you to practise.

- The final stage involves the internalisation of the energy being shifted inside you. Now the bodily movements become quiet, the external manifestations of the spinal movements are almost invisible and the Chong Mai is fully opened up. This means that you have reached a high level in your Dao Yin training. It is now likely that you will experience the soft white glow in your head as the Shen is raised up through the Chong Mai.

The process outlined in this chapter covers the higher level energetic stages that can be achieved through practice of the Dragon Dao Yin exercises. You have moved beyond the physical bodywork of opening up the joints and connecting the Jing Jin together, and into the energetic realm of shifting Qi through the various branches of the Chong Mai. This reflects the movement from physicality through to energy work, which is inherent in all Daoist internal arts. For the final part of this work I wish to discuss the stages of progressing beyond here into the realm of Nei Dan, Daoist alchemy. The Dragon Dao Yin exercises can serve to form a way into the higher level, meditational practices of this ancient tradition through a process known as 'Lighting the Lower Cauldron'.

MOVING INTO NEI DAN

So far we have looked at the process of working to clear the energy body of stuck pathogenic energy in order to build the foundation for more advanced training. The energetic processes of working with Kan and Li inside the body as well as 'Waking up the Dragon' have been discussed, which are the first stages in moving Dao Yin training towards the more advanced levels of practice. In this final chapter of the book an overview of Nei Dan is given. Nei Dan is often translated into English as 'internal alchemy' and it is probably the best known form of Daoist meditation. Though a complete discussion of Nei Dan would take up an entire book or two on its own, it is worth looking at the process of Daoist Nei Dan in order to understand how it works. The reason for this is because any form of energetic exercise from within the Daoist tradition can serve as a doorway into Nei Dan practice once it has been trained in for long enough. The Dragon Dao Yin are no exception to this rule and those who engage with the more advanced stages of Dao Yin practice outlined in this book may find that they begin to move naturally into the processes outlined in this chapter.

The first thing to understand is the different definitions of Qi Gong, Dao Yin, Nei Gong and Nei Dan. Each teacher will define these terms slightly differently, according to how they were taught and their own understanding, but for the purposes of my own work this is how I personally use the terms:

- **Qi Gong:** Qi Gong can be translated as 'energy work'. It usually takes the form of static or moving postures combined with a particular intention and breathing method. Most Qi Gong exercises tend to have a particular function; they are aimed towards a specific goal. These goals may be directed towards improving health, martial power or any one of a number of other benefits. Although they may take the form of a life study and they can take a person very deep into the internal world, they do not have a transformational process inherent within them.

- **Dao Yin:** Dao Yin exercises are the moving, stretching exercises discussed in this book. They aim to purge the body of stagnant energies and so are primarily aimed at improving a person's psychological and physical health, although they can also be used for developing martial skill. For a full discussion of the differences between Qi Gong and Dao Yin please refer back to the first chapter of this book.

- **Nei Gong:** Nei Gong is a process rather than a specific set of exercises. Translated as 'internal skill' or 'internal development', Nei Gong uses different tools to move a person along a particular line of internal development. The tools used are a mixture of breathing exercises, sitting practices and Qi Gong routines. The Nei Gong process focuses initially upon awakening a practitioner's normally dormant energy system via direct accessing of the lower Dan Tien. Further stages involve generating strong internal energetic movement along the lines of the meridian system and then beginning the conversion of vital substances inside the body.

- **Nei Dan:** Nei Dan is the alchemical process of refining the base essences of a person's internal environment in order to refine the quality of their internal energy and develop the nature of their consciousness. The practitioner's consciousness is raised to such a state that they return to the original point of stillness from which they were born and experience direct connection with Dao. This is the meditation process most commonly associated with the Daoist tradition, although some Daoist schools use different meditation practices.

It becomes complicated once we begin to look at how these practices relate to each other. They almost form a sequential process that a person could follow, but not quite, due to the amount of overlap they have with each other. Figure 8.1 shows the relationship between the different practices.

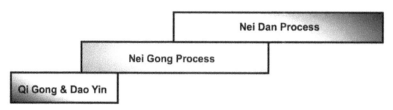

FIGURE 8.1: PRACTICE RELATIONSHIPS

As you can see from the diagram, Qi Gong and Dao Yin form the foundation practices. They are a start point for anybody wishing to move into Daoism, but they will only lead to the earliest levels of development possible through Nei Gong training. These low levels of attainment are often struck upon accidentally through Qi Gong and Dao Yin training, which can be surprising to those practising these arts. The Nei Gong process can take a person deep into the internal arts, but not as deep as Nei Dan can. There is a strong overlap between Nei Gong and Nei Dan but ultimately there is a glass ceiling which will never be passed if a practitioner does not engage with the meditation practices of the Daoist tradition. It is an interesting aspect of Daoism that it combines energetic practices with meditation, whereas many other wisdom traditions focus solely upon one or the other. It is also often the case that people will have a preference for one or the other. In the West I have met many who like energy work but do not have the patience for meditation, and vice versa. Daoism requires a person to engage with both energy work and meditation, due to the close connection it has between Qi and Shen, energy and spirit.

Please note that I do not seek to offend any Qi Gong practitioners by stating that it does not go as deep as Nei Gong. Remember that these are only according to my definitions as I was taught them. Perhaps your definitions are different from mine? According to my understanding of the terms I believe that many who say they are practising Qi Gong are actually practising Nei Gong, and the same is true in reverse. It is the process contained in any system that takes a person deep into Daoism, not the external exercises.

The Dragon Dao Yins are a good example of how a practice can begin to lead a person through the sequence of development shown in Figure 8.1. This is because they develop as you spend more time practising them. At the beginning you learn the various movements and go through the process of adding in the different layers of energetic detail which transform them into full Dao Yin exercises. At this stage you are working in the foundation stages of the above developmental sequence. This changes when you reach the stage of standing and 'Waking up the Dragon' at the end of each of the four forms. This process which you have engaged with begins to change the way in which Qi flows in the congenital meridians; it activates the lower Dan Tien and starts a deep internal process. At this time you have moved into the stage of practising Nei Gong. The Dragon Dao Yin exercises are no longer simply medical exercises with a specific goal; they have progressed to the point of leading you through a deep process of internal change. Transformation is unfolding within you and the Nei Gong process is being worked through; the exercises have become tools for this process. Once there has been a certain degree of movement through the length of the Chong Mai it is possible to start touching upon some of the earliest stages of the Nei Dan process. In particular the stage of 'Lighting the Cauldron' which sets the stage for further alchemical change.

THE BASIC PREMISE OF NEI DAN

Nei Dan is based upon the theory that all of existence was formed from consciousness. From the still point of Dao, original spirit is born and this is known as a form of Shen. Shen then slows down or condenses to form Qi, the basis of the energetic realm. From here there is a further process of transformation and Jing or essence is formed. This gives birth to the physical body, and in this way human life comes into being. The gradual slowing down or condensing of these substances known classically as the 'Three Internal Treasures' takes place in us through the function of the three Dan Tien, which act as a way of 'stepping down' frequencies in the body during our developmental process. Figure 8.2 shows this process.

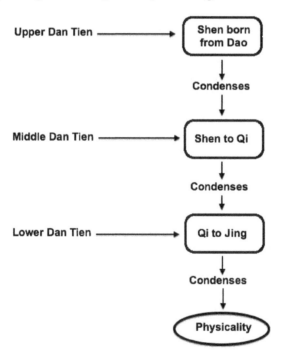

FIGURE 8.2: THE PROCESS OF INTERNAL CREATION

For a more complete discussion of this process please refer to my previous books through Singing Dragon.[1] This process continues until we have a complete physical form, which ultimately reaches its conclusion upon our birth. From here it continues to unfold to a lesser degree as movement across this process actually begins to take place in both directions; from Shen to Jing and from Jing to Shen. As we age and move through adolescence, the downward movement from Jing to Shen begins to move into the background until we are eventually functioning almost entirely according to the second process, shown in Figure 8.3.

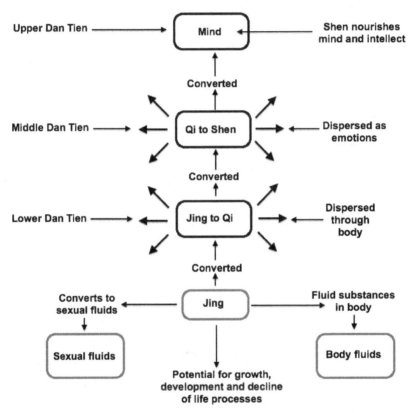

FIGURE 8.3: THE ACQUIRED MOVEMENT OF JING, QI AND SHEN

Though it may be a slight oversimplification of what is taking place in us it is a useful model to work to when we first begin to move into alchemical training such as Nei Dan.

1   Mitchell, D. (2011) *Daoist Nei Gong: The Philosophical Art of Change*. London: Singing Dragon and Mitchell, D. (2013) *Heavenly Streams: Meridian Theory in Nei Gong*. London: Singing Dragon.

The foundation for the movement and transformation of the Three Internal Treasures begins, in this process, with Jing. Note that Jing in this diagram does not reside in the lower Dan Tien. This can often cause confusion. The job of the lower Dan Tien is simply to convert Jing into Qi. The Jing itself does not reside in the lower Dan Tien, it instead sits between the Kidneys near to the Mingmen (DU 4) acupuncture point. This is the storehouse of original essence which was given to you at the point of your birth. Your Jing is used up over the course of your life through several different processes which are discussed below. As your Jing declines, you begin to move through the ageing process until you reach death.

In many contemporary Qi Gong schools Jing has been equated solely with sexual fluids. This is simply not the case. Jing is the potential for physicality but it is not physicality itself. Jing, Qi and Shen are simply forms of vibrating information which sit 'behind' the physical realm. They form the basis for tangible existence but they are not existence itself. Essentially they are one and the same. Jing, Qi and Shen are the frequency range beyond that which we can usually access through the realm of the five senses. They take different forms, depending upon which frequency range they are operating within. The ease of transformation between the Three Treasures is because of their ultimate one-ness. If we raise the frequency of Jing it transforms into Qi and then further into Shen. If we lower the frequency of Shen it transforms into Qi and then lower again converts it into Jing. When Jing decreases further in frequency it manifests on a physical level and gives birth to form. Within the external environment the slowing of Jing creates matter, whilst within the internal environment of the human body Jing will turn into one of several substances, sexual fluid being just one of these substances.

From Figure 8.3 we can see that Jing, which sits around the area of the Mingmen acupuncture point between the Kidneys, gradually gives birth to the various fluids in our body. These fluids include all of the substances which give us life, including Blood, which is formed in part from Jing and in part from our Qi. These substances are essential to our life processes. Jing also governs the state of our physical body and dictates exactly how fast it moves along the ageing process. All processes of growth, development and decline which our physical body go through are dependent upon the state and relative amount of our Jing. If we do not take care of our essence then we will age faster and the health of our physical body will fail. In this way we can understand our Jing as being like fuel of which we have only a certain amount. It is for this reason that Jing is often translated into English as 'essence'. Anybody who has studied even the most elementary level of Chinese medical theory will know that Jing is seen as very important. Guarding against its decline is a major part of both Chinese medical and Qi

Gong theory and, since the Kidneys are seen as the storehouse of the Jing, they are considered very important to look after.

The Jing that is stored within the area of the Kidneys also produces sexual fluids in both men and women. This essence travels down to the area of the perineum at an acupuncture point called Huiyin (Ren 1), which means 'meeting point of Yin'. This area of the body controls the sexual fluids. In classical Chinese medical thought the amount and quality of Jing in this region also governs the level of your libido (in conjunction with the Yang aspect of the Kidneys) and your fertility levels. In the West there is often an attitude of 'more is better' with regard to sex. Our society is set up to encourage this aspect of human desire and there is little understanding of the effects this has upon your health. According to Chinese medical thought, the more we use up our sexual fluids, the more our Jing is forced to produce, which means that through sex we are gradually depleting our essence. This speeds up the ageing process as well as weakening the body, as the Jing plays a large part in dictating our physical constitution; in particular, the health of the lower spine and knees is closely related to the level of our Jing, so chronic long-term pain in both the back and knees is almost always attributed to a weakness in our Jing.

This understanding of loss of Jing through use of sexual fluids often causes a great deal of concern amongst those who study Chinese medicine or the Daoist arts. In particular it is often a concern for male students, as most of the damage to a person's Jing is the result of external ejaculation, something that is not such an issue for women. Whilst sexual intercourse still depletes the Jing of women, it is such a tiny level of depletion that it is hardly a risk. It is much more depleting for men. The study of how to minimise this loss is long and complex, as celibacy is not recommended by the majority of Daoist sects, being seen as unnatural. Instead certain practices developed which would help with preservation of Jing, but a discussion of these practices is beyond the scope of this book. For those studying any form of internal art it is worth simply sticking to the principle of moderation. If you have either a weak back and knees after having sex, or you are finding that directly after sex you wish to fall asleep, then you are over-depleting your Jing. Sex should leave a person feeling refreshed, energised and positive, otherwise it is a sign that Jing levels are declining. Celibacy is required for certain stages in the Nei Gong process but only for periods of time, as discussed below. Any longer periods of celibacy combined with internal practices should take place under the supervision of a qualified teacher.

The final way in which Jing is used up is through its conversion into Qi. The Jing from the Kidneys passes into the lower Dan Tien region which converts it into Qi, which is then distributed throughout the body. This Qi is vital for the functioning of every aspect of your existence, as all of your internal organs require this vital energy to maintain their functional activities. This conversion from Jing into Qi is the primary way in which Jing is used up. The Qi converted from your Jing is combined with Qi drawn from food and air to make up the vital energy we use in the course of our daily lives.

The Qi that is not dispersed through the body into the organs is then converted upwards once more via the energy of the middle Dan Tien into Shen, which is the energy of our consciousness. Much of this spiritual energy is used up as we experience our shifting emotional states, and that which is left moves upwards into the upper Dan Tien which sits in the centre of the brain. This Shen contributes to our intellect and the forming of our acquired mind.

Though many of the more intricate stages involved in the conversion of Jing to Qi to Shen are not included in the above description, it is sufficient for us to be able to understand exactly how we use up our Jing and how our body functions throughout our lives. The speed at which we age and die depends mainly upon how we treat our bodies and how well we look after our Jing.

A note here has to be made of the differences for women. The above description discusses the way in which Jing, Qi and Shen move in a male body. Women do not lose their essence to the same degree through intercourse but instead lose it through menstruation. Consequently many systems of Daoism developed a practice known as 'Cutting the Red Dragon' which essentially means stopping menstruation so that Jing is not lost each month. This would be the female Daoist equivalent of complete celibacy for men, and ultimately it is a risky and unnatural process. I have met many women who have engaged in this training and the vast majority of those who have done it for some time experience great health problems. What is often misunderstood is that menstruation is supposed to take place, as it is also cleansing in nature. Women's energy naturally moves deeper *into* the body than men's, which tends to move outwards. This is the key Yin and Yang energetic difference between the genders. As male energy expands outwards it naturally cleanses a certain amount of internal toxins, whereas women's energy does not; their cleansing takes place during menstruation over the course of four or five days. If menstruation is deliberately stopped then this cleansing mechanism is ended and internal stagnation can take place. This stagnation can lead to fertility problems and serious diseases in later life. The problem with 'Cutting the Red Dragon' is that those who originally practised it were renunciates. They lived away from society and basically had a life that revolved 100 per cent around their internal cultivation. Close monitoring of their health was maintained by a master and toxins from the environment were minimised through clean air, minimal social contact and healthy living. It would have been very different from attempting such methods whilst living in modern society where your mind and body are constantly under attack from external pathogens. It is a fool's game to attempt advanced practices intended for reclusive living whilst leading a 'regular' lifestyle. It is better to guard the health of your Kidneys and follow a healthy lifestyle in order to protect your Jing.

TRANSFORMING YOUR JING, QI AND SHEN CYCLE

Through the early stages of Nei Dan, which can also be accessed through Nei Gong training, it is possible to change the way in which the Jing, Qi and Shen cycle takes place in your body. The change in the above process means that Jing, Qi and Shen move as shown in the diagram in Figure 8.4.

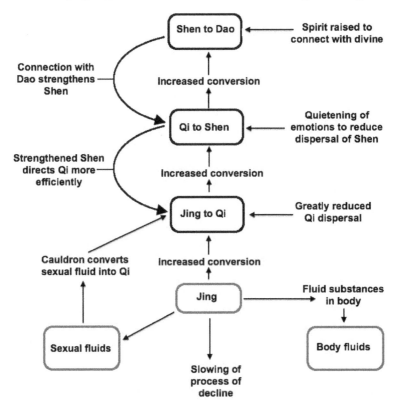

FIGURE 8.4: THE NEI DAN CYCLE

In this version of the process of internal change between Jing, Qi and Shen there is less wastage of any of the Three Treasures through dispersal. When looking at the process of Jing converting into substances we can see that it has changed. The conversion of Jing into fluids is pretty much the same; it is possible to change this to some degree but it actually takes place at much later stages in Nei Dan training. This primarily concerns changing the nature of our Blood but it is not relevant to the foundation stages of alchemy practice. The overall movement of our Qi and Shen through the body, combined with healthy living, slows the ageing process as the Jing is recycled through the system. The sexual fluids, which are stored at the base of our perineum, change and are no longer simply built up ready to be lost through ejaculation. Instead the Lower Cauldron, which is discussed below, actually enables some of this sexual fluid to be converted 'upwards' into Qi, which then moves through the system. In this way Jing, which would have been lost through intercourse, now adds to the overall health of our body and the energetic circulation of the meridian system. This is a major way of slowing the depletion of Jing and a strong form of internal medicine.

As the Jing moves into the lower Dan Tien to be converted into Qi it is strengthened by the extra energy created by the conversion of the sexual fluids back into Qi. The work done on the lower Dan Tien reduces the amount of Qi dispersal from this region as it flows more efficiently through the meridian system. As the Qi moves up into the middle Dan Tien to be converted to Shen this can happen more effectively as less is dispersed by the emotions, which should have been brought more under the practitioner's control. This is one of the key reasons for the importance of governing the emotional mind in alchemical schools. The practice of the Dragon Dao Yins should have helped to purge pathogenic energies created by excessive emotional states. This helps to break the cycle of emotional imbalance, which helps in bringing the emotional mind under control. In this way the Dao Yin training in this book has been setting the foundations for further development through the Nei Dan process. The extra refinement of Shen taking place as a result of reducing dispersal from the middle Dan Tien enables it to be raised up towards the upper Dan Tien, where it is possible, through prolonged practice, to convert it further upwards to the frequency of Dao itself. This brings connection with the divine and profound insight associated with high-level internal cultivation practices.

The cyclical nature of Daoism then takes this process further. The higher we can raise our Shen, the more effectively we are able to guide our internal energy, and so our Qi flow becomes stronger. Thus the effects of prolonged Nei Dan training through this process are cumulative. Through practices such as the 'small water wheels of Qi' discussed earlier we add to this recycling of the Three Treasures, and so the depletion of essential substances is greatly reduced. This slows the ageing process, improves health and enables the Three Internal Treasures of Jing, Qi and Shen to be focused towards cultivation practices.

THE DRAGON DAO YIN EXERCISES AND NEI DAN

Much of the work required to engage fully with the Nei Dan process takes place from a seated position, as is common for most forms of meditation. That said, the early stages of Nei Dan, and in particular the process of Lighting the Lower Cauldron, can actually begin through other energetic practices such as the Dragon Dao Yin exercises, once a high enough level has been reached. This is because of the overlapping nature of the different practices, as represented in Figure 8.1. It is too easy a trap to fall into to associate a particular practice with a particular result. Many practitioners falsely believe that each internal method they learn will lead to only one very specific outcome but this is really not the case. There is an internal process of development which the body and mind can be taken through during training of the internal arts; as we progress we move through the various stages. All exercises we work on will move us through this process, even the most simple and basic exercises that we may have learnt when we were beginners. It is just that some methods are more efficient than others for certain achievements. That is why, when I write my books, I often include information on the stages of internal development that traditionally come at a later stage than the processes outlined in the book. Experience has shown me that many students actually stumble upon more advanced stages than they would expect to reach through the exercises they are working on, simply because they have sufficiently prepared their energetic system and this enables it to evolve of its own accord.

Once the Chong Mai has been opened, the Dan Tien is awakened and much of the energetic stagnation from the meridian system has been cleared it is likely that you will have prepared the energy body sufficiently for Lighting the Lower Cauldron. When the energy body is ready, it is common for the Cauldron to 'light' on its own and the process of moving into Nei Dan to begin naturally. As far as I am aware this is as far as you will be able to progress, though, as any further internal development will require training in the seated alchemical practices of Nei Dan. The advantage of Lighting the Lower Cauldron is that the way in which your Jing, Qi and Shen moves will start to transform between the two cycles discussed above. This helps to preserve Jing, efficiently cycle Qi and raise Shen towards the upper Dan Tien. It is the beginning of the creation of the 'internal elixir' discussed in Daoists texts. This is a miraculous form of internally created medicine which nourishes the body and rejuvenates the tissues.

WHAT IS THE LOWER CAULDRON?

The Lower Cauldron is one aspect of the lower Dan Tien. As well as rotating to send Qi moving through the congenital meridians of the body, the lower Dan Tien raises the vibration frequency of a person's Jing to help convert it into Qi. When the Lower Cauldron 'lights' it causes this to happen more efficiently, resulting in the transition from A to B as shown in Figure 8.5.

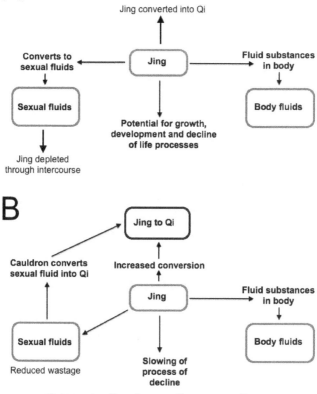

FIGURE 8.5: THE LOWER CAULDRON FUNCTION

The key change that takes place in the lower Dan Tien is that it begins to have a direct relationship with the point which controls the build-up of sexual fluids. This is the Huiyin (Ren 1) point, which sits at your perineum. As the Dan Tien and this point begin to function together as one unit, there is a change in the way that your sexual fluid moves and much of it is recycled up into the energy body, converting it into Qi. This is essential energy which would otherwise have been depleted through sexual activity. Doing this does not reduce fertility. It is important to make this clear, as there are often many fears around this kind of work. Rather, it transforms any excess sexual energy that builds up around the perineum. Remember that according to ancient Daoist thought the direct connection between essence, energy and mind means that the build-up of sexual fluid around the perineum also dictates the state of a person's mind. For example, if a person does not have sex for a period of time, perhaps several weeks, it is normal for their desire for sex to increase. Particularly for men this can be a real issue. When teaching it is common for me to advise students to decrease their sexual activity. For training purposes it is not wise for males to have sex every day, and this of course includes masturbation. Teaching a great many people has shown me that it is quite normal for many men to have sex or to masturbate at least once per day. This is far too much and depletes the Jing which we require for our internal work. Daily ejaculation will make it impossible to build a strong foundation in the internal arts. As students lower their sexual activity in order to help strengthen their Jing they usually experience a desire for sex, which makes it very difficult for them. According to Chinese medical thought this would not just be their biological instinct kicking in but also a result of the build-up of sexual energy around the perineum area as the Jing continues to convert down into this area. When we 'light' the Lower Cauldron the need for self-control is lessened somewhat, as the excess build-up in this region is reduced. The sexual fluids convert upwards into Qi and the desire for sex decreases to a healthy level. It is normal for any questions of 'How often should I have sex?' to become irrelevant at this stage, as the body will know what is right. Instinctual understanding will replace biological desire and in this way the energy body will regulate itself naturally.

When the Lower Cauldron 'lights' it is normal for the heat in the region of the lower Dan Tien to expand downwards towards the perineum. The whole region of the pelvis becomes warm, as well as the area of the Kidneys. This is not a temporary warmth such as is experienced in some other developmental stages in the internal arts. This warmth will stay, no matter what the outside temperature, so that when somebody touches your lower back or abdomen they will feel that it is warm to the touch.

Traditionally it was a skill that had to be demonstrated by meditating in the snow, so that it was clear to a practitioner's teacher that they had achieved the Lighting of the Lower Cauldron. Along with this you will also feel a 'bubbling' sensation around the area of the perineum. When you feel this it is easy to see why the ancient Daoists used the term 'Lower Cauldron' for this process. It feels much like bubbling water that is radiating heat around the lower abdominal region. This bubbling is the conversion of the sexual fluids building up around the region of the perineum. These converted substances are then refined into Qi, which moves back into the energetic system to be cycled through the meridians. This process is not just limited to men; many of the processes in Nei Dan can differ greatly between the sexes, but the Lighting of the Lower Cauldron is not specific to male practitioners. It is only after this stage that the Nei Dan process differs for women.

As this recycled energy moves into the body it increases the quality of the energy moving through the meridians. This is greatly rejuvenating for those who reach this stage. The following reactions result from the Lighting of the Lower Cauldron:

- As the increased flow of Qi moves through the system it is normal to experience increased energy levels. Any chronic feelings of exhaustion, which many people live with, fade away, leaving a person feeling rejuvenated. Children prior to puberty function all of the time in this state, provided that they are healthy, and so your energy levels will begin to return to the way they were when you were a child.

- The increased Qi flow combined with the decreased loss of Jing results in a person needing less sleep. It is normal to be able to function well on fewer hours' sleep than you previously required. The amount of hours you need will depend upon how effectively the Cauldron has been lit. During prolonged Nei Dan retreats it is normal for students to be able to reduce their sleep to around three hours, as the Lower Cauldron is working very efficiently.

- As the refined Internal Treasures move upwards in the energy system they help to settle the emotions and bring mental clarity. Thought processes become sharper and your mind seems to function at a higher level than before. There is less mental clouding, so that you can function more effectively on a daily basis.

- Your immune system will usually become stronger and it is possible to shake off imbalances in the body. Many chronic sicknesses can disappear at this stage, especially if they were conditions based around 'deficiency' according to classical Chinese medical thought. This is the result of the internal medicine being produced from wtihin the body once it is able to reduce Jing leakage and increase Qi production and circulation. In China it is more common for meditation to be known as a form of healing than it is in the West, and for the Daoists it was the process of Lighting the Lower Cauldron that they were aiming for in order to experience the medical benefits of Nei Dan.

Once the Lower Cauldron is lit it is wise to spend some time each day just standing and observing it take place. Breathe deeply and just 'listen' to what your body is doing. Giving the process this internal space to unfold will help it to become natural for the body and gradually it will become a permanent way for your energy body to function. Be warned, though – the increased energy levels can make you feel 'on top of the world' but you must still exercise caution. When I first reached this stage I was amazed at just how much energy I had. My drive was greatly increased and my mind was far more focused. Consequently I embarked upon a period of working myself to my limits. I spent all day each day pushing myself and enjoying the benefits of this increased energy, only to reach a point where I basically collapsed! I had drained my essence through overwork and it took me some time to repair the damage I had done. Enjoy the benefits of this process but still remember that you are not superhuman, no matter how you feel. Preserve your energy and take a longer view of your well-being than I did.

FUELLING THE LOWER CAULDRON

When the Lower Cauldron first 'lights' up it is normal to experience the warmth and bubbling sensations described above. If you wish to capitalise on this attainment and 'fuel the fire' then it is useful to store your Jing as much as possible. This is one of those stages where temporary abstinence from sexual activity can be useful. Classically the guideline for this was to stop all sexual activity for 100 days or three months. If you reach the stage where the Lower Cauldron is 'lit' then it should be fairly easy to complete this length of abstinence. The three months of no sexual activity will enable all of the Jing moving into the perineum region to be converted up into Qi, and in three months the internal medicine connected to this stage is complete. This will fully nourish the body and complete the foundation required for further alchemical training in Nei Dan. During this time, if you spend an hour or so each day focusing upon what is taking place in the body then sexual desire will fade, making the three months an easy thing to complete. For many students it can normally be difficult to abstain from sexual activity for this length of time, but once the Lower Cauldron is 'lit' it is not difficult at all. The conversion of the Jing into Qi dissolves any sexual desires. If these desires do not fade then it is likely that the Lower Cauldron is not ready and you have not reached the required stage in your training just yet.

For many this can be a powerful form of internal medicine for clearing the mind and repairing health. Building this foundation also makes progression in any of the internal arts much easier. It helps to fully transform the way your body works energetically. It will be the natural function of the energy body to raise the frequency of Jing to Qi to Shen, provided that you continue to train in the internal arts and maintain your health. It will make progression through any internal arts much faster and more efficient, as your energetic system will adapt to the new practice much faster than it would have done before. Your emotional state will also centre to a large degree, making you less prone to swings between extreme emotional states. An interesting benefit for those who previously found that their thoughts were taken up with sexual desires is that they will lessen. The common belief that men think of sex every few minutes/ seconds no longer applies, as the mind is more able to focus without being based solely in the physical desires.

CONCLUDING THOUGHTS

When I write, I like to make sure that I only really discuss any internal processes that I have experienced for myself. In this way I wish to ensure that I don't go down the road of teaching Daoism from a purely intellectual standpoint. I believe that Daoism is more of an experiential art than a cognitive one and that anybody teaching it, either through verbal instruction or written guidelines, should be able to give you the benefit of their own tangible experiences. For this reason I am limited as to how far I can explain some processes by the limits of my own internal development. As far as I am aware this is about as far as exercises such as the Dragon Dao Yins can take you. They can help to clear out the energy system, free up emotional stagnation, condition the body, open the Qi Men, awaken the energy of the spine and Light the Lower Cauldron. Any work beyond this must be completed through other exercises, such as Nei Dan training. To be perfectly honest, though, I think that the above processes that Dao Yin training takes you through are pretty far-reaching! By the time a practitioner has reached these stages they have moved quite deep into the internal arts. If you were to start these exercises from scratch with little or no prior experience of the internal arts, it would take a number of years of dedicated practice in order to work through the stages of development outlined in this book.

It is my hope that those reading this book have been able to see how Dao Yin training differs from Qi Gong training. I also hope that I have explained adequately what the function of Dao Yin exercises are is and how they can be used to purge the energy body of negative energies. If I have explained either of these inadequately then I apologise, perhaps it is wisest to practise them for yourselves so that you can actually feel the differences between the two systems.

Any book like this is very difficult to write, especially as I am not an experienced writer. I had never even tried to write anything before I worked on my first Nei Gong book. It is difficult for me because I am trying to take classical teachings which I have studied for a long time and combine these with sensations and experiences to be had through following these teachings. Often these sensations are very difficult to put into words, so that possibly only those who have already shared these experiences will actually understand what I am talking about! Another difficulty is that one person's experience may differ from another person's, so that ultimately the experiences written here are very subjective in nature. I have considered this and wondered whether it is best to just stick to facts and leave out any personal experiences or opinions, but then I believe that many other books already do this. Consequently I feel that it is best to take the experiences from this book and make a note of them, train in the exercises and keep an eye out for similar experiences, but at the same time do not fixate on them. The reason for this is because your experience may be different. Sensations just depend upon how your brain translates the information associated with the energetic process you are going through; though there will likely be similarities, there will also likely be subtle differences personal to your own development.

This is my third book published through Singing Dragon. *Daoist Nei Gong: The Philosophical Art of Change* outlined the Nei Gong process and the fundamental principles common to all internal arts, whilst *Heavenly Streams: Meridian Theory in Nei Gong* looked at the medicinal nature of Daoist work and the meridian system. I feel that the previous two books, along with this one, form a trilogy which covers a lot of the foundation knowledge required for understanding the Daoist internal arts as I see them.

At the time of writing I have been involved in the Eastern arts for just over 29 years. The first ten of these years were focused solely upon bodywork through practices such as Indian yoga and the external martial arts. From here I moved into the internal Chinese styles and then progressively into Chinese medical practices, Nei Gong and Nei Dan. My practice has developed along the somewhat classical path of being interested in combat, through to medicine, through to spiritual growth, and now Nei Dan is the main focus of my practice. Though each day I sit and work on raising Shen to illuminate the third eye and connect with Dao, I never neglect bodywork practices such as Dao Yin.

As you move deeper into your practice, the spaces of time between clear signs of progress become wider. Whereas the early stages of development saw regular improvements on an almost weekly basis, the more advanced stages see these clear developmental milestones being divided by years or more. Faith in the effectiveness of the practice is your training companion, as diligent perseverance is required, even in the face of little developmental encouragement. Often I have found that in order to help this progress along it is wise to return to the basics. When struggling to understand the far reach of your own stage of attainment it is often beneficial to go right back to the root of what you are doing. This is seeking to elevate Yang through engaging with Yin. Sometimes I have been trying to work with a subtle aspect of the spirit and failing miserably, but as soon as I returned to Dao Yin training the 'penny dropped' and I was able to increase the limits of my ability. In many ways I feel that this is the biggest strength of the Dragon Dao Yin exercises. Though basic in comparison to a practice such as Nei Dan, they are profound in their ability to help you progress in your spiritual cultivation.

Perhaps one of the greatest strengths of Daoism is the interconnected nature of their practices. When Shen cannot be altered, change Jing or Qi and allow Shen to change of its own accord. This is how I use the Dragon Dao Yin sequences and for this reason I believe them to be a relevant practice at any stage on your journey towards union. I hope that others reading this book will also find them of use, from the beginner seeking to relax his or her body through to the advanced alchemist one step from attaining the golden light body of immortality. I have had a lot of fun and benefit from my practice of the Dragon Dao Yin and I hope that I have managed to explain their theory and practice adequately so that others may gain the same.

About the Author

Damo Mitchell was born into a family of martial artists and so began his training at the age of four. This training has continued throughout his life and expanded to include the study of martial arts, meditation and various forms of Chinese medicine, as well as Nei Gong. His studies continue to take him around the world in search of authentic masters of the ancient wisdom traditions which he teaches through his own school, Lotus Nei Gong, which has branches in the UK, Sweden and the US.

Damo continues to spend his time travelling, teaching, writing and studying around the globe. For more information on Damo and where he is teaching, please refer to his website: www.lotusneigong.com.

GLOSSARY OF PINYIN TERMS

In this glossary simplified Chinese characters have been included for reference purposes, except where traditional Chinese characters are still commonly used, as in the case of Chinese medical terminology.

BAGUAZHANG 八卦掌 A Chinese internal martial art based on the eight trigrams of the Yi Jing.

BAIHUI 百會 (DU 20) An acupuncture point situated on top of the head. Translated as meaning 'hundred meetings'. In classical Daoism it is also the point where numerous spirits converge and the point where the Chong Mai extends upwards out of the body.

CHONG MAI 衝脈 The most important meridian within the congenital energetic system. The central branch of the Chong Mai runs straight through the core of the body, between two points known as Hui Yin and Bai Hui.

CHUANG TZU 莊子 An ancient Chinese work from the late Warring States period (3rd century BC). One of the two foundational texts of Daoism, along with the Dao De Jing.

DA ZHOU TIAN 大周天 'Large heavenly cycle', also known as the large water wheel of Qi. This is the primary circulation of energy out of the body which can be achieved through consistent alchemy or Nei Gong training.

DAN TIEN 丹田 Usually refers to the lowest of the three main 'elixir fields'. Its primary function is the conversion of Jing to Qi and moving the Qi throughout the meridian system.

DAO 道 The nameless and formless origin of the universe. Daoism is the study of this obscure concept and all internal arts are a way of experientially understanding the nature of Dao.

DAO DE JING 德道经 The 'the virtue of following the way'. The classical text of Daoism written by the great sage Laozi (see below). Also written as *Tao Te Ching*.

DAO YIN 導引 'Guiding and pulling exercises.' These are the ancient exercises developed by the shamanic Wu people to purge the energy body of pathogenic energies.

DE 德 The congenital manifestation of the transient emotions. De is born from deep in the true human consciousness which is usually buried beneath the various layers of the Ego.

DUI 兌 One of the eight trigrams of Daoist Bagua theory. Its energetic manifestation is metaphorically likened to a lake although Dui does not directly mean lake.

FA JIN 發勁 This is the external expression of an internal energy. It is issued from the core of the body and emphasises body connection.

FENG SHUI 风水 'Wind and water.' This is the Daoist study of environmental energies and the influence of the macrocosm upon the human energy system and consciousness.

GEN 艮 One of the eight trigrams of Daoist Bagua theory. Its energetic manifestation is likened to that of a mountain.

GUA 卦 'Trigram.' These are the eight sacred symbols which make up Daoist Bagua theory. They are a way to conceptualise the various vibrational frequencies of the energetic realm and how they interact.

GUANYUAN 關元 (Ren 4) An acupuncture point located underneath the navel. Guanyuan governs sexual functions. It is also used in treating menstrual disorders.

HUANG DI NEI JING 黄帝內經 An ancient Chinese medical text that constitutes the main authority for practitioners of Chinese medicine.

HOU TIAN 後天 The acquired or 'post-heaven' aspect of our nature.

HUIYIN 會陰 (CV 1) 'Meeting of Yin' is an acupuncture point located at the perineum. It is named after the fact that it is situated in the most Yin area of the human body.

HUN 魂 'Yang soul.' The ethereal soul which continues to exist after our death. It is usually housed within the liver.

JI BEN QI GONG 基本气功 'Fundamental energy exercises.' The primary exercises taught in the Lotus Nei Gong School of internal art.

JIANJING 肩井 (GB 21) Point located on the shoulder. Helps with stagnation and tightness in the area of the shoulders.

JING 精 The lowest vibrational frequency of the three main energetic substances of man. Usually translated as meaning 'essence' and often misunderstood as being human sexual fluids.

JING GONG 精功 'Essence exercises.' The technique of building up and refining our Jing.

JING LUO 经络 The human meridian system which is made up of numerous energetic pathways that regulate the body and transport Qi to and from our organs and tissues.

KAN 坎 One of the eight trigrams of Daoist Bagua theory which is usually likened to the energetic manifestation of water.

KUN 坤 One of the eight trigrams of Daoist Bagua theory. Its energetic manifestation is usually likened to that of the planet.

LAOGONG 劳宫 (PC 8) An acupuncture point situated in the centre of the palm. Its name means 'palace of toil' due to it being on the human hand which carries out a lot of physical work. In Daoism they also know this point to be very important in venting heat from the heart and so it is rarely at rest. Very important point in Qi Gong practice as it regulates the internal temperature and also allows us to emit Qi in practices such as external Qi therapy.

LAOZI 老子 The great sage. The original Daoist who wrote the *Dao De Jing*. Supposedly he left this text with a border watchmen when he retreated into hermitage in the western mountains of China.

LI 離 One of the eight trigrams of Daoist Bagua theory. Its energetic manifestation is usually likened to fire.

LONG DAO YIN 龍導引 'Dragon Dao Yin.' A set of four sequences based upon the preliminary training methods from the martial style of Baguazhang. They twist the spine and open the joints to assist with the energetic purging process.

MING 命 Your predestined journey from life to death. Usually translated as meaning 'fate' but this really does not explain the true meaning of the term.

MINGMEN 命门 (GV 4) An acupuncture point in the lower back which is very important in Nei Gong practice. This point is referred to several times in this book and serious internal arts practitioners should work very hard to awaken the energy in this area of their meridian system.

NEI GONG 內功 The process of internal change and development which a person may go through if they practise the internal arts to a high level.

PI FU 皮肤 The layer of skin that surrounds the entire body and exists as the outermost layer of the physical body. It constitutes the external barrier between our inner body and the external environment.

PO 魄 The 'Yin soul' which dies with the human body. Largely connected to our physical sense; the Po resides in the lungs.

QI 氣 'Energy.' A term that is often difficult to translate into English. In Nei Gong theory it is an energetic vibration which transports information through the energy system.

QI GONG 氣功 Usually gentle exercises which combine rhythmic movements with breathing exercises to shift Qi through the body. The term means 'energy exercises' although it is sometimes translated as meaning 'breathing exercises'.

QI HAI 氣海 (CV 6) An acupuncture point which sits in front of the lower Dan Tien. Its name in English means 'sea of Qi' as it is the point from where Qi is generated and where it flows from. Like water returning to the sea in rivers and streams, Qi returns to the lower Dan Tien when it circulates in the 'small water wheels of Qi'.

QI MEN 氣門 The main energy gates of the body.

QIAN 乾 One of the eight trigrams of Daoist Bagua theory. Its energetic manifestation is usually likened to the movements of Heaven.

REN 人 In Daoism, Ren is 'humanity'. Humanity sits between Heaven and Earth and is a reflection of their fluctuations and movements. Ren is nourished by Earth and stimulated to development through Heaven.

SHANGZHONG 膻中 (Ren 17) An acupuncture point located in the middle of the chest. It corresponds to the heart centre.

SHEN 神 The energy of consciousness. Vibrates at a frequency close to that of Heaven. It is manifested in the body as a bright white light.

SHEN GONG 神功 This is the arcane skill of working with the substance of consciousness. In Daoism it is said that a skilled Shen Gong practitioner can manipulate the very energy of the environment.

SHU POINTS 俞腧穴 These are points located on the back, on either side of the spine. They are standard points used in acupuncture treatments.

SISHENCONG POINTS 四神聰 Four points located on top of the head. They are often used in cases of possession.

SUN 巽 One of the eight trigrams of Daoist Bagua theory. Its energetic manifestation is usually likened to that of the wind.

Sung 松 This is the process of transferring habitual tension from the physical or consciousness body into the energetic realm where it can be dissolved.

Taiji 太极 A Daoist concept of creation which can be translated as meaning the 'motive force of creation'.

Tian 天 'Heaven.' Not to be mistaken for the Christian concept of Heaven; this refers to the vibrational frequency of the macrocosm. In the microcosm of the body Heaven is used metaphorically to refer to human consciousness.

Tiantu 天突 (Ren 22) An acupuncture point situated at the base of the throat. Can be used to release pressure in the chest.

Tui Na 推拿 A form of Chinese medical massage which means 'push and grasp'.

Wu Xing 五行 The five elemental energies which are an important part of Daoist creation theory, psychology and medicine.

Wei Qi 衛氣 A protective energetic layer that guards us against invading pathogens and emotional information.

Wu Xing Qi Gong 五行气功 'Five Element energy exercises.' They are an important part of the Lotus Nei Gong syllabus.

Wuji 无极 The Daoist concept of non-existence. The blank canvas upon which reality is projected and an important part of Daoist creation philosophy.

Xian Tian 先天 The congenital or 'pre-Heaven' aspect of our nature.

Xin-Yi 心意 'Heart-Mind.' This is the framework with which we attempt to understand the various aspects of human consciousness. Originally a Buddhist concept, it was absorbed into Daoist teachings.

Xingyiquan 形意拳 A Chinese internal martial art that focuses on developing intention.

Xuan Men 玄門 The Xuan Men or 'mysterious pass' describes the point when the three bodies of Man (physical, energy and consciousness) fall into perfect balance.

Yang Qi 阳氣 Our internal Qi which moves out towards the surface of the body and the congenital meridians.

Yang Shen Fa 养身法 Literally, 'life nourishing principles'. This is the Daoist practice of living healthily which should be studied alongside all internal arts.

YI 意 'Intention' or 'awareness'. An important element of human consciousness to cultivate in Nei Gong training.

YI JING 易经 The 'Classic of Change'. An ancient Daoist text which is based upon Bagua theory. Commonly written as *I Ching*.

YIN QI 阴氣 Our internal Qi which moves in to nourish the organs of the body.

YONGQUAN 涌泉 (K 1) An acupuncture point on the base of the foot which means 'bubbling spring'. This is the main point through which Earth energy is drawn into the body.

ZANG FU 脏腑 The collective name for the Yin and Yang organs of the body.

ZHEN 震 One of the eight trigrams of Daoist Bagua theory. Its energetic manifestation is often likened to thunder.

ZHI 志 An element of human consciousness which is directly linked to the state of our Kidneys. The nearest translation in English is 'will power'.

ZHONGFU 中府 (LU 1) This is a 'window of Heaven' point that allows you to access the spirit of the Lungs.

ZIRAN 自然 The Daoist philosophical concept of acting in harmony with nature and returning to an original state.

APPENDIX

MERIDIAN POINTS REFERRED TO IN THE BOOK

A number of meridian points have been mentioned throughout this book. These are shown on the diagram below. For more detailed descriptions of their location and functions please refer to any good acupuncture textbook.

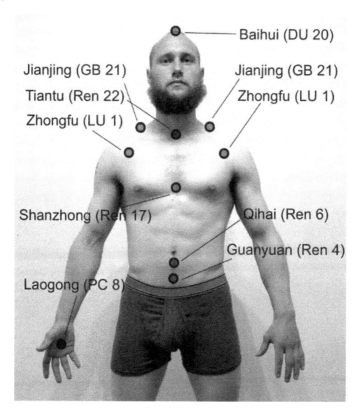

Baihui (DU 20)

Jianjing (GB 21)

Tiantu (Ren 22)

Zhongfu (LU 1)

Jianjing (GB 21)

Zhongfu (LU 1)

Shanzhong (Ren 17)

Qihai (Ren 6)

Guanyuan (Ren 4)

Laogong (PC 8)

247

INDEX